Beyond Metabolism

How Your Brain, Biology and the Environment Create and Perpetuate Weight Issues ...and What You Can Do About It

by Scott Abel

Published by:

Scott Abel

ISBN-13: 978-1514195697
ISBN-10: 1514195690

Table of Contents

Section Two
Solutions

About the Author

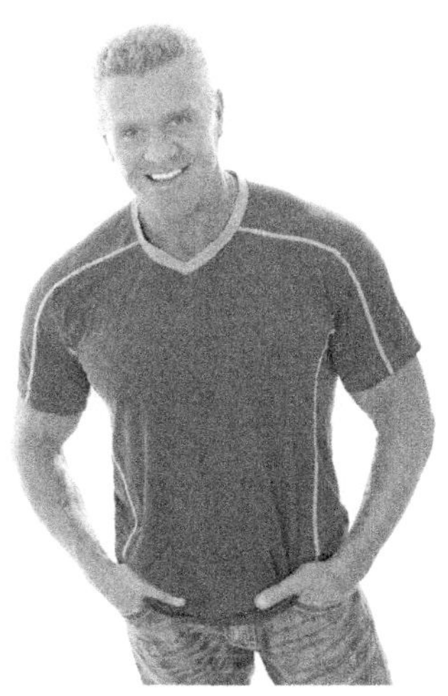

Scott Abel has been involved in the diet, fitness, and bodybuilding industries for over four decades. His coaching specializes in physique transformation rooted in a mindset for longterm success.

This book is about your environment, your habits, and weight control and weight loss. The first section is about the biological and cultural factors that have "overridden" the wisdom of the body, and what causes unnatural, irresistible cravings, weight issues, and food issues.

The second section is about *solutions*.

Introduction

I spent over thirty years studying nutrition and diet, but up until the past few years I only researched these topics in the most accepted and conventional ways. In the last decade however, I learned a valuable lesson—the usual way we approach diet and nutrition is wrong.

This is why countless people search for diet and eating solutions in all the wrong places. They attack their issues symptomatically instead of causally, and this just makes things worse. If they only address the *real* causes of their struggles and perceived failures, they can succeed on their diets, eliminate food-related anxiety, and adopt effective dietary habits.

Many experts have written on this in terms of the biology of weight control, but far fewer have written about it with respect to the brain and our habits. That's where this book comes in.

"You Are What You Eat" (...sort of)

Everyone has heard the expression, "You are what you eat."

I've known many coaches who parrot the expression to clients who find it difficult to stick to a diet.

Many of my own clients have heard me turn this phrase upside down and say, "As much as you are what you eat, your issues with diet are about *what's eating you.*"

But even this statement is incomplete. The truth of the modern diet situation is this:

You are <u>what</u> you eat.

You are <u>how</u> you eat.

You are <u>why</u> you eat.

With this in mind, **if we all know "what" to eat, why don't we just do it?**

We know what foods are healthy and we know what to avoid. We know more about nutrition than at any other time in our history. And if we listen closely to our bodies we also know how much food is too much.

So where is all the food and diet stress coming from?

Why is there so much diet confusion?

Why can't we stop snacking?

Why can't we stick to a diet?

Confusion About "Diet"

The shelves of any bookstore are filled with books about diets and dieting. No other animal on the planet needs to be told what, when, why or how to eat, how to eat, and neither did we, until recently.

From internet gurus to lifestyle magazines to The Biggest Loser we are shamed, scolded and humiliated by proclamations that we need to extremely restrict our caloric intake in order to lose those unwanted, unsightly pounds, and are weak if we cannot comply. On the other side of that brittle coin, we are told by zealous vegans to eschew any animal product, by passionate paleo-dieters to eschew grain, by low-carbers to never let a grain of rice pass our lips. The truth is, with a protein shake, a multi-vitamin and a diet of Twinkies you can lose substantial weight and improve your blood lipid profile (as Dr. Mark Haub did), though I don't advocate eating high-reward, addictive junk in order to control your weight.

Perusing the aisles of my local bookstore recently, it struck me that nearly all of the books are written about the diet itself—what, when, where, why and how you should eat. But we're smarter than that, aren't we? Deep down you know there is no magic diet. True victory over food and weight issues is not about the diet. It's about the dieter—**you**.

It's always been about you.

When you look at evolution, you'll find that human survival was based on key neural developments and adaptations that made for a sharper mind. Like most animals, we pursue pleasure and avoid pain. The psychology of diet that comes with our evolved brain is now at odds with a world of modern food abundance and food stimuli.

In this book, we will examine how some people become susceptible to food or diet influences that eventually dominate their life. You will discover how your own brain is affected by our modern environment. By addressing your brain, habits and environment you will overcome your weight and food issues. We will uncover the elements that "magic diets" fail to address, and highlight the underlying operating system you need in order for any diet to truly "work." This is not about nutrient timing or any other complex diet regimen.

I will mention throughout this book **one important message:**

Almost all of these issues we will address are about the "dieter."

...and they are *non*-metabolic issues.

Many issues we'll look at *affect* your metabolism over the long-term, but they are not intrinsically metabolic. The underlying issues—the ones we need to address—have to do with your brain and your environment.

Abundant research suggests that modern food stimulates the reward circuits of the brain, driving people to overeat. The food industry has capitalized on this research to create and sell more and more indulgent foods. By contrast, the diet and fitness industries seem to ignore the research. Many fitness professionals will say you just need more willpower. The concept that you **"lack willpower"** is a tremendously damaging and false pronouncement that you may have experienced firsthand.

One of my clients, for instance, developed an eating disorder induced by her previous competition dieting strategies. She'd initially reached out to her former coach, confessing that she was unable to stick to her diet. She described what she was going through both physically and mentally. Her coach told her: "Champions don't cheat on their diets."

Micromanaging diets, nutrient composition and so on, are not solutions our food and diet issues but rather diet prisons we create for ourselves. Food and diet issues are psychological, biological and neurological issues. They are *seldom* metabolic issues.

Portion control and calorie counting result in short-term weight loss that invariably lead to long-term weight and food issues. This short-term fix causes long-term problems.

Psychology and Biology

What is important to understand and embrace is this:

"Thought determines the experience of behaviour."

Look at the key words in the phrase:

- "**Thought**" refers to the *mental* elements preceding behaviour.
- "**Experience**" refers to the *emotional* consequences of that specific behaviour.
- "**Behaviour**" refers to the actual *physical* act.

The **mental**, **emotional**, and **physical** elements of being are what I refer to as the 'triangle of awareness.' When discussing food issues, it's impossible to effectively address one area without addressing the others, yet the diet industry has been doing just this for decades.

We need to stop looking at food and diet issues as external, objective solutions to problems that are more complex and multi-layered. A 'diet' is simply the object in the equation. The **subject** of the equation is *you.* How many diet books or diet articles have you read that talk about **you**—your experiences, feelings or thoughts?

If thought determines the experience of behaviour, you have to address the thought and the experience. Your own personal and individual mindset and feelings regarding diet, food and weight are subjective elements to understanding your modern diet or food issues. These subjective elements are being ignored, when they are actually the key components of the solution.

The combination of the biology of weight control **(physical)**, personal experience and history **(emotional)**, and the billion-dollar food, diet and supplement industries **(environmental)** all contribute to our food, diet and weight issues. Everyone's diet dilemma will be unique, based on varying degrees of influence and individual characteristics. For people with very sensitive metabolic set-points, for instance, a single diet to lose weight can be a catalyst for a *lifetime* of food, eating, diet and weight issues.

Some of the environmental stimuli accosting us at every turn include:

- The prevalence of food
- Larger portion sizes
- Endless selections of specifically engineered, hyper-palatable tastes and textures
- Convenience of food
- Marketing of food as reward

When we combine these with our present-day attitudes of entitlement and desire for immediate gratification, it's easy to understand how any food issue can spiral out of control.

"Indulgence"

I have chosen the word "**indulgence**" to encapsulate the modern diet dilemma.

- For the **physical** component of the equation I refer to "indulgent foods," such as those which have unnaturally high levels of salt, sugar, fat or various combinations of each. These foods cater directly to the reward center of the brain and are engineered to do so.

- For the **emotional** component I use the term "indulgent food/diet issues" because the term outlines over-*thinking*, over-*reacting* (instead of responding) or over-*feeling* your diet and food stress.

For the **behavioural** element, I you'll see the same term as above: "indulgent food (or diet or eating) issues," meaning actions or *behaviours* such as overeating excessive eating, starving and bingeing—the actual "act" of eating (or not eating), in other words.

Over the decades I've seen that it's the psychological issues that influence my clients' abilities to adhere or not to adhere to a diet. Every year clients approach me with diet and body-image stresses that have, over time, led to indulgent food issues. These people have gone from one solution to the next, one diet to the next, one guru to the next, forever believing that the next diet, or the next workout program, or the next expert, is the solution to their food issues.

This is why food *denial* and *deprivation* are just as indulgent as overeating. There is an incredible similarity between people who mindlessly overeat and those who overanalyze every morsel that passes their lips. People suffering from anorexia will deny food, but the term "indulgence" as I am using it still applies because food and diet preoccupy the anorexic's mind to a physically and emotionally debilitating level. Less extreme but just as relevant, dozens of men and women I've worked with, who boast enviable physiques, were miserable because of their indulgent thinking about food. The weight issues may not always show but that doesn't meant people aren't suffering. Thoughts of food dominate their lives and destroy their self-esteem.

A harsh truth is that some people choose to suffer and don't even know it.

But another truth is that no one has to suffer from indulgent food issues. There are solutions. You can regain control of your eating, your brain and your habits.

The remedy is not so much about conquering these issues as it is about learning how to let them go with practiced awareness. But know that awareness has many levels within itself. There is no finite end, but a fathomless depth to grasp and put to good use, one discovery at a time.

With that in mind, let's move on to the questionnaire.

You, the Dieter
A Questionnaire

Self-understanding is a large part of the awareness we are seeking in order to solve our diet dilemmas. So for this questionnaire, record your answers, but more importantly, have a notebook and a pen handy to write down whatever thoughts you have about any points that particularly apply to your personal experience. If any of these questions cause a physical reaction, make a note of it.

Some points will feel extremely personal, whereas others won't apply at all. That's fine. Everyone experiences food issues differently. Only you have the answers to your own dilemma.

Since I first released this questionnaire, I've received a lot of feedback. People have told me that when they reviewed their answers they cried. It can be eye-opening and hard to face some of these truths. But it's important.

Go into it with an open mind, and be brutally honest.

(Note: you can download a formatted, printable version of this questionnaire, with room for personal notes at scottabelfitness.com/foodquestions.)

Questionnaire:

1. Are your waking thoughts consumed or dominated by issues that deal with how you eat, why you eat, resisting the urge to eat, or equating any of the above to how you feel about yourself?
2. Is food or diet never far from your conscious mind?
3. When you think about yourself and food, do you think in absolute terms of being either "on" or "off" a diet or eating regimen?
4. Are you easily distracted or even upset by having indulgent food (goodies) in your presence?
5. Do you have an emotional conception of right and wrong foods? Do you eat the 'wrong' foods only when alone, and/or do you hide your eating of indulgent foods?
6. Do you always know more or less exactly what you weigh?
7. Do you ever find yourself eating indulgent foods even when you know at the time you really don't want to?
8. Do you ever participate in post-indulgent guilt

practices like 'guilt-cardio' the day after an indulgence, or cutting carbs and restricting food the day after an indulgence?

9. When it comes to indulgent eating do you find yourself arguing internally with yourself, before or after?

10. Do you feel powerless around indulgent foods, especially specific kinds of indulgent foods?

11. When indulgent food is present at (for example) a staff meeting or somewhere you do not expect it, and not at meal times, do you spend time or focus on that food in a sensory way? In other words do you focus or get distracted by how good it looks or smells?

12. Does the scenario in question 11 cause you to react emotionally and try to resist the temptation of eating or even noticing the food? (Or do you merely see it as there for others, but do not 'feel' it at all?)

13. Address honestly how you respond to a food cue. If your favourite food is put in front of you, do you find it hard to resist even if you are not hungry? Does such a scenario create an inner struggle?

14. Do you wake up each day and start a battle of 'food is my enemy'?

15. Do you find yourself more than once per day engaging in self-talk or emotional reaction

regarding food or diet?

16. Do you stick to a diet for a few days then always blow it?

17. Do you have a difficult time knowing when you are full or satiated?

18. Do you feel remorse, shame or guilt after a diet sabotage? If so, rate that emotional state on a scale of 1-10, 10 being the highest.

19. Do you rationalize unwise eating choices or food denial choices in strange ways? If so, do you engage in psychological negotiation with yourself about it?

20. If you consider yourself overweight, skip this question. If you are thin do you stay that way only because you wage a constant mental and emotional battle within yourself about food, each and every day?

21. Do you consider yourself 'not thin' or 'not lean' and therefore do you hate or despise your body or certain parts of it because of this?

22. Are you preoccupied about what you are going to eat or how much exercise you need to do to burn it off? Are you emotionally attached and attracted to workouts advertised as "fat-burning," "fat torching" or "fat melting?"

23. Do you get angry at yourself over how much time you spend thinking about food or diet?

24. If someone says something hurtful to you, do you

often react by thinking about or taking part in a food indulgence?

25. Similarly, if you have a bad day do you find yourself reacting to this by thinking about or taking part in a food indulgence?

26. Do you find yourself tired or even exhausted over your inner emotional reactions to your thoughts and feelings about food/diet/weight? In other words do the related feelings of fear, guilt, anger, shame, exhaust you?

27. Do you ever dream about food?

28. Do your preoccupations with food focus on foods you like and want, or on foods you try to avoid? Are any of these foods the same?

29. Do you equate being alone with being lonely?

30. When you are alone do you try to find something to do to occupy yourself?

31. Is alone time a danger time for you to either overindulge or obsess about resisting food?

32. Will you go out of your way to pursue a food reward? Would you impulsively drive to a store to buy an indulgent food you crave, or plan an indulgent food procuring outing?

33. Do you always know what you weigh?

34. Does the weight scale itself create an emotional reaction in you? Is the scale a source of fear, dread or reward? Do you give the scale the power

to dictate your mood?

I hope you have taken the time to not only answer these questions, but think about them as well in the most personal and intimate sense. Using these questions as a starting point can not only teach you about yourself but also pinpoint your problems within the triangle of food and diet awareness.

I have deliberately spread these questions out and not grouped them in sections. But all of these questions, taken together, address the physical, mental and emotional elements of food, diet, weight, and your own *experience* of food, diet and weight.

What have you learned from this questionnaire?

If you think it hasn't told you anything you don't already know, then look again. Address this questionnaire as a scale of intensity. In terms of answers, **the more questions to which you answered yes, the deeper and more extensive your issues with food, eating, and weight are.**

Step 1:

Count the number of "yes" answers.

If you answered "yes" to 4 or more questions you have some sort of food, eating or bodyweight issue that is negatively impacting your life. What you need to address is to what degree this is true for you.

Step 2:

After answering 'yes' to any of these questions, then rate them in terms of intensity on a scale of one to ten.

As you address yourself by answering these questions, look also at the the diet/fitness/supplement industry. If you have any of these issues, emotional, mental, physical, and behavioural, **has a diet or nutritional knowledge ever done anything to solve or cure your issues?**

It's time to get real.

The diet industry has no stake in anyone actually solving these issues.

To solve any of these issues is to disassociate food from the conscious process of thought and emotion. No matter how externally successful you think a diet is, if you are still over-concerned with food, you're not holistically healthy. Only when food and diet become non-issues; only when you have more important things to think about are you free from your diet-prison.

In assessing the results from this questionnaire, I find that there are three constants at work either separately or combined, to varying degrees:

- People feel a loss of control regarding indulgent foods.

- People feel unsatisfied by food they expect should satisfy them.

There is some kind of overriding preoccupation with food and diets.

Your relationship with food is a reflection of your relationship with yourself and with life but a"diet" does not define you. It is not part of you, but rather something you 'do to yourself.' If you refer to yourself as fat, ugly, weak, etc., your actions, behaviours and emotions around food will play out as a self-fulfilling prophecy.

Section One. Your Brain, Your Body, and the Biology of Weight Control

Chapter 1. The Real Biology of Weight Control

If you're thinking about long-term health (or long-term weight loss) you must understand and work with the biology of weight control. There are very specific biological mechanisms in place for modern man that simply cannot be ignored.

Promises of a "revved up metabolism" or "easy weight loss" or "hunger-free fat loss" are lies created by an industry that panders to desire and vanity. **For many of you dreaming of a new sculpted body, this chapter may not be what you *want* to hear, but it's exactly what you *need* to hear!**

The Modern Day: What Changed?

For millennia, the average human body weight stayed

remarkably stable. Most people naturally ate about the same amount of calories they burned off. Things were good. There were very few people who were overweight.

The 1980s saw several far-reaching monumental shifts in our attitudes toward food, and in our food supply. Dietary fat was singled out as the most villainous culprit responsible for weight gain and declining health. The food industry adjusted by replacing saturated animal fats with "heart healthy," super-processed vegetable seed oils, and high fructose corn syrup. Soon, our average body weight started to rise, and it did so quickly.

- In 1960, when bodyweight was stable in North America, women ages twenty to twenty-nine weighed roughly 128 pounds.
- By the year 2000, the average weight of women in the same age group reached 157 pounds.

Population studies show a trend that is beyond individual weight control. Children now enter adulthood at higher and higher body weights and the trend continues to increase. Weight margins are increasing across the board at every age of human development.

Here's the thing: the biology of weight control explains this phenomenon quite well. When you factor in the biology of weight control, instead of those numbers being shocking or baffling, they become understandable. The question is not one of metabolism, as the diet industry would like you to believe. Our metabolisms aren't changing. So then, what we need to know is which lifestyle drivers are now present, and which have become absent, in a way that would influence the weight trends we're seeing. What lifestyle drivers could cause such changes when for millennia bodyweight stayed stable?

Physical labour is no longer woven into our day-to-day lives. I'm not talking about the Industrial Revolution. I'm talking about recent changes. The 1950s "housewife" worked a staggering sixteen hours per day, six days a week. This was physical labour by today's standards. The amount of calorie-burning movement required to cook meals, wash dishes, clean the house, do laundry (all without many of our modern conveniences) is something people of our generation cannot relate to—even if we *think* we can.

People from the 1930s to the late 1950s did not formally exercise because their daily lives included large amounts of physically demanding exercise. This part of the calories-in, calories-out equation is absent from our present-day lifestyle. But changes in the amount of physical labour is only a small part of the biology of weight control.

In terms of human evolution, we have evolved to embrace weight gain. Randy Seeley, a neuroscientist at the University of Cincinnati puts it this way:

> "Your body wants to be fat. Getting fat is what it is supposed to do. And trying to persuade your body not to be fat is going against everything the body is designed to do."

We are designed to fight famine, weight loss, muscle loss and catabolic states, all in order to deal with periods of less available food.

James Hill, director of Colorado Clinical Nutrition Research Unit says, "Humans have only a very weak physiological mechanism to defend against weight gain when food is abundant, and yet very many safeguards to defend the body against weight loss." When confronted with abundance, our bodies do the exact opposite of what we want them to do.

As we will see in upcoming chapters regarding the human brain, man pursues food as reward as a matter of survival. It is a primary biological drive, just as it is with other animals.

What we know about the human biology of weight control not only accurately explains the rate of weight gain in modern society, it predicts it as well. The upregulation of bodyweight set points I mentioned above is predictable given the modern environment of food abundance, food convenience, extra time available for food indulgence and an instinctual drive that seeks food as a reward.

Conceptually, this element of the biology of weight control has been labelled the "absence of protection" model. The absence of protection model suggests that being overweight results from a biological system that was never designed to work in a world of limitless food, so we have no protections against it. If somehow we *had* evolved in a world of abundance, we probably *would* have those protections, just as we have protections against famine (something our species actually dealt with).

One explanation I've discussed often is that when leptin (a hormone) levels fall *below* a certain threshold, the body recognizes this as a signal to build up a storehouse of energy; it is a biological response to caloric deprivation. (Whether you call it "a diet" or starvation is incidental. Your body doesn't know the difference.) But the opposite effect does not occur—when leptin levels rise there is no predisposition to lose weight.

Disruption of Hunger and Satiety Feedback Loops

What this means in plain language is that food intake rather than energy expenditure (exercise) is the main factor responsible for weight gain.

Dr. Lee Kaplan, MD, PhD and Director of the Massachusetts General Hospital Weight Center, said this when he spoke at Harvard Medical school:

> "There is a central regulatory system. The body is very good at matching energy intake and energy expenditure to a very close tolerance. The tolerance is about .15% averaged on a daily basis. The mechanism by which this process of balancing food intake and energy expenditure occurs is a simple biofeedback controlled by parts of the brain. If you decrease your energy intake so that you lose weight arbitrarily, you will become hungrier so that you return energy intake to a higher level. If you arbitrarily try to gain weight, the opposite will occur. The epidemic of obesity is not divorced from this system; the epidemic of obesity is a disruption of this system. It's not McDonalds only; it's McDonalds as it disrupts this system. It's not your genes only. It's your genes as they affect the balance of this system."

I see Dr. Kaplan's thesis play out all the time in my practice, in terms of climbing bodyweight set points that directly result from dieting.

I've witnessed this effect with my physique competitor clients my entire career.

The very nature of competing in figure competitions requires incredibly strict dieting for prolonged periods, without a break. Among physique competitors, over 75% typically weigh more and look heavier than they did before they began contest prep. This is especially prevalent in female competitors. Women who started in the low to mid-120s gain twenty to thirty or more pounds within two years. Many of them rationalize this as "lean muscle" gain. It's not.

Dozens of studies illustrate Dr. Kaplan's point. The processes dictating appetite and hunger are tightly regulated. They are also, as we are finding out, easily disrupted. Depending on genetics, a single ill-advised diet can put someone on a path to permanent, frustrating weight gain.

Metabolic Compensation

Metabolic compensation is the unconscious, biological adjustment of calorie intake over a period of a day or several days that ends up balancing out to a consistent level of caloric intake. If you deprive yourself for a few days, your body's mechanisms will, in response, trigger hunger and eating cues to bring you back to normal.

What disrupts this system and leads to unwanted weight gain is sustained deprivation diets. People who engage in extreme or frequent diets (physique competitors for example) often lose the capacity to gauge their hunger or fullness. Once this happens the balancing mechanism—metabolic compensation—is not only disrupted, but broken.

A broken metabolic compensation system leads to climbing body weights. (No, it doesn't really work the other way. You can't "break it" to pre-dispose yourself towards weight loss, at least not to the same degree that you can break it and pre-dispose a body towards weight gain.)

Conversely, research has also shown that people can gain weight with *as little as 25 extra calories per day* once their compensation systems are disrupted. This is the equivalent of one single small apple once every three days. Clearly the consequence of short term dieting can be dire long-term. The problem is that our metabolic compensation system gets affected over the long-term, but our modern day diet and weight "studies" and ubiquitous success stories littering the media landscape utilize a narrow window.

The body is smarter than the mind. Evolution has made us that way. We focus on twelve-week transformations, before-and-after photos and fitness models on magazine covers. But when looking at calorie compensation *long-term,* it balances out. Of course magazine covers don't show that.

Dr. Friedman, a molecular biologist, determined that

energy intake and expenditure over a decade falls within .17% percent—perfectly balanced. You are not going to fool your body long-term, even though you may disrupt its perfection. Every calorie you deprive your body of in the absolute sense (i.e., with an extreme diet) will be balanced and restored down the road, but the 'disruption' part of your body's metabolic compensation system means this restoration and balance works out to unwanted higher set points and body weights. Call it caloric karma if you like.

In Dr. Friedman's words: "this [compensation system] exceeds by several orders of magnitude the ability of nutritionists to count calories!"

Metabolic homeostasis is under sustained assault because of modern convenience and, in turn, our misguided attempts to override the wisdom of the body.

Hunger

The concept and feeling of hunger has been not only disrupted but warped in the current climate of indulgence. The introduction of snacking, resulting from the food industry's influence has distorted the gut's perception of tolerable hunger.

Constant snacking, plus our perception of hunger as an unpleasant state that requires immediate relief makes it so that our modern eating behaviours lack conscious awareness. Conversely, or subsequently, the same eating behaviours claim far too great an emotional attachment. Following a restrictive diet only intensifies our reactive behaviours.

In truth, a certain degree of hunger should be considered a natural state.

Tolerable hunger keeps satiety reflexes operating as they should. A degree of hunger is the natural state of all animals, especially predatory animals. (And human beings are predatory animals.) Hunger is a primary source of our survival drive. It is not unnatural—if anything, fullness beyond satiation is unnatural. Culture and industry have turned the biology and societally accepted perception of hunger upside down.

Various environmental influences and even memories can underlie susceptibility to unhealthy food indulgences or diet habits. Both unsatisfying moods and unsatisfying meals can lead to further eating or becoming preoccupied with food. There is a huge difference in gut and emotional response to the myriad levels of hunger. There is also an entirely different biological response between being ravenously hungry and "noticeably" hungry. The metabolic patterning and compensation involved with both of these works itself out for better or worse over time. So in real terms of the biology of weight control, a diet based on caloric deprivation alone without regard to individual subjective biofeedback, can predict heavier body weight trends long-term.

Exercise

I see it all the time—people adding more and more activity thinking it allows them to eat more and more.

While it all *seems* to work in the numbers they crunch in their online fitness trackers, things seldom work out in terms of sustained weight control. Whether you overeat in huge single sittings or snack your way there, overeating has the same result over time. You cannot out-train an unbalanced or incorrect diet.

Physical activity levels are not good predictors of weight control, regardless of what is marketed to you. (And yes, this is also true of strenuous exercise and the overly hyped EPOC of workout intensity—see *Modern Nutrition in Health and Disease*, 10th edition, p. 8).

* * *

It is not the timing of carbs or types of fats that have this or that effect on leanness. These complicated strategies are but a small part of the story. I do admit that such practices may have some validity on the metabolic elements of dieting, but very little regarding the biology of simple weight control.

If there is a single truth to take away from this chapter it is this: *how much* you eat predicts how much you will weigh, not *what* you eat (barring any preexisting medical conditions of course).

In terms of the biology of weight control the principle of Occam's razor applies. Do you really think your increasing weight is due to a lack of understanding these super intricate elements of diet, carb-timing, and complicated caloric formulas? No, all things being equal, the simplest explanation tends to be the right one. People weigh more because they eat more.

Chapter 2.
Your Brain's Reward System

Contrary to the diet and fitness industry's emphasis on weight control via this or that diet, there is much more at work here than calories-in/calories-out, metabolism, or even the biology of weight control discussed in the previous chapter.

This is because there is always an **interplay** between your **mind**, your **emotions**, your **environment**, and your physical responses.

There is no separation in terms of this "triangle of awareness." Biology acts *on* and *with* mental and emotional neural influences. Each of these elements can affect the others, consciously or unconsciously. When you try to isolate one element you come up short.

Learning to study the difference between high carb or low carb diets only gives you a myopic view of what's at stake. This kind of understanding won't explain your own eating behaviour, or the patterns and habits you adopt; it will never enhance your own awareness.

The human animal is wired to pursue both momentary *and* long-term rewards. For instance, sex not only satisfies an immediate need; it also serves to perpetuate the species. The food drive works the same way. Early humans evolved the ability to respond to environmental cues that led to the rewards they sought, Our ancestors became cognitively and emotionally aware of their surroundings and in this way, obtained their mates and their food, thus ensuring our existence today.

A cue is anything that can trigger and stimulate your thoughts and emotions and hold your attention: a sight, a smell, a sound, a thought, a feeling. This can *all* take place unconsciously.

To this day we respond to environmental cues, mentally, physically and emotionally. If you were to see a food label, say, advertising the logo of your favourite ice cream, you would experience signs of physical hunger. Perhaps as well you might think back to a time when you enjoyed ice cream with your family on a summer day, or you might find yourself flooded with guilt or anxiety.

Since environmental stimuli play such a huge role in our decision-making, what we need to cultivate is a healthy level of conscious awareness when it comes to our oftentimes unconscious and unhealthy responses.

"Survival of the fittest" was guaranteed by our adaptability and a cognitive ability to learn from environmental stimuli. Humans learned how to develop a focus on the most significant stimuli in their environment. This could mean fleeing from a predator, pursuing prey, or pursuing a mate.

In the present-day landscape of food abundance, cues abound, and we're wired to pay attention to them even when we'd clearly be better served by ignoring them. Yet this "drive for food" is innate. And so is appetite.

Commanding Our Attention

Food has the power to command our attention both in pursuit of it, and in the experience of it. For modern humans the experience of food is especially important.

We know that humans evolved to pay particular attention to any cues for food availability. This attention leads to a certain level of psychological and physiological arousal. This level of arousal is directly tied to both biological hunger and psychological appetite.

A Reverse Pavlovian Example

I feed my dog at the same time every day. Within minutes of that time his attention focuses on his impending meal, and he lets me know it is almost time to eat with excited anticipation. The process of me getting his dish is one environmental cue that sets in motion his emotional awareness of an anticipated food experience.

The reverse is also true. For the *rest* of the day, even in the presence of food, he does not respond in

the same way at all unless I introduce certain other cues. He has been conditioned to focus on food only at a certain time of day, and *not* focus on it at other times.

It's not that different for humans.

A rewarding food experience usually will involve sight, smell, texture, and even a memory associated with a previous positive food experience. Emotionally rewarding responses to a food cue can become not just powerful, but totally overpowering. The most effective rewards are the ones that alter feelings. When food takes on that power, it gains much more emotional reward value than it would in nature.

For people who are more susceptible to this type of emotional influence, food cues become the new stimulus to attention-bias. Indulgent eating or a desire to do so is the natural emotional response to this.

Commercials can initiate the arousal response in the brain. A certain day of the week, like "Pizza night" Fridays, or nachos during Sunday football can also trigger this response. These and many other cues can act as invitations to the brain. Each cue is based on previous emotionally rewarding food experiences. Your vulnerability to an emotional food cue doesn't disappear because it is a learned and conditioned response.

Because of the reward center of the brain, rewarding foods, whatever that may be for you personally, tend to become reinforcing events. They are in the truest sense of the word, "comfort foods," in terms of the emotional effect they have.

The danger here is that the sensory layering of a food experience can mean that other stimuli can also become conditioned and internalized as being associated with certain foods. The other stimuli may not even be food-related, yet by association still trigger an emotional arousal and desire for that food.

Pavlov's dog salivated upon being presented with his food before eating it. This was his natural physiological response. Then he was presented his food along with the ringing of a bell. This action was repeated until the mere sound of the bell was enough to cause the dog to salivate.

But how many of you have associated this kind of classical conditioning to the abundance of food cues in our modern world? This is what is happening. It is as though different bells of all shapes, sizes, and tones, are ringing and ringing and ringing. Our brains receive the signals, and we salivate for more and more and more. You could no more stop that dog from salivating at the sound of the bell by simply telling him to stop, than you could stop yourself from eating an indulgent food just by telling yourself oh, don't think about eating that food so much.

What are the bells that arouse these responses in your own head?

Cognitive Association

The association between a given food and a pleasurable experience is what's known as a **"cognitive association."**

This is one of many ways, for instance, that McDonald's becomes part of the social fabric: you remember going there as a kid. Similarly, there is a reason food brands want to be associated with pop culture events. It's not purely about the taste (though the hyper-palatability plays its own important role), but about the association between a particular food and a *seemingly* non-food-related experience.

Remember at this point that the taste of the food itself is only one small component of the overall rewarding 'experience' associated with that food indulgence.

This is extremely important to understand, and explains how certain cultures also respond to specific food cues. You may grow up to crave pasta because that was your family Sunday meal when you were a kid. For others, that association may be roast beef, or Friday-night pizza, or any number of other cognitive food associations.

Stimulating the brain with associated food experiences provides a sense of momentary pleasure, and possibly even escape. In today's environment this type of escape can become problematic when it masks deeper, more painful emotions. But since the brain focuses on anticipation and desire for a pleasurable experience, emotional eating results.

Conversely, emotional *resistance*, in denying or resisting a certain food by constantly thinking about it, is really still the same issue playing itself out in the opposite direction.

The Fix Doesn't Last

When you eat for pleasure you create a brief moment where you experience reward or relief. The cognitive association for the food-fix may have been reinforced over a period of years, but it provides only a moment of pleasure. You end up wanting to achieve that emotional state again, much like a drug addict anticipating that next line of cocaine.

Not only are there far more food reward cues than ever before, but the cues also have *greater intensity*, in terms of commanding our awareness and attention. The palatability, taste and texture of processed foods, for example, are more immediately gratifying than whole natural food. This means that the psychological lure of food is far more intense as well.

One study showed that animals will actually work for the rewards of foods high in sugar and fat, even if they are not hungry. How hard animals will work for this reward is similar to that of addicts seeking out cocaine. Modern discovery of sugar and sweeteners as well as fats to add texture to food has increased palatability, and the intensity of the experience it provides. The more rewarding the food experience becomes the more habitual and intense will be our pursuit of it.

As if the chemically manipulated food were not enough, we are also confronted with relentless advertising, strip malls, restaurants and entire television networks devoted to food, all designed to further influence our brains toward food pursuit as an emotional reward. These super-stimulating foods and food-cues create increased levels of hunger and appetite. None of this is actual metabolic or biological hunger. The intensely increased palatability levels of modern food capitalize on the ancestral parts of the reward system of the brain.

It is natural for us to pursue good-tasting, emotionally satisfying foods; it is wired into our brains to do so. What is not natural is the new levels of taste experience which push the experience level far beyond satisfaction to a level close to drug addiction.

Variety

Once upon a time, coffee was served black, or with cream and/or sugar. Modern coffee comes caffeinated, decaffeinated, half-caff, blond, medium or dark roast, espresso blend, fair trade, organic, hazelnut, vanilla, and if you're not living under a rock, you could list dozens of additional varieties without pausing.

Then there's the cream—dairy, non-dairy, heavy, light, half-n-half, soy, coconut, and of course so many flavours. Imagine telling someone from the early 1900s that they could choose from twelve kinds of cream, let alone twenty different types of coffee. Imagine their face staring up at a Starbucks menu. Frappucino. Americano. Salted caramel half-caf soy latte with an extra shot. Pumpkin spice. Peppermint mocha .Which one would he or she like? They wouldn't know where to begin.

Coffee is just one tiny example of the powerful level of influence variety and palatability have in stimulating the reward centers of our brains, and we haven't even mentioned the grocery stores! We simply have not yet evolved to handle the infinite availability, palatability and variety of food offerings.

Food reward patterns in your brain are permanent

Once these neural patterns for reward through food experience are established in our brains, they never disappear.

Ever.

Even after someone overcomes their food, eating and diet issues, the stimulus-response sequence can re-emerge.. Using food as a pleasurable distraction in times of stress—even once—can cause food, diet and eating issues to begin all over again.

The connection between a cue and a memory is never completely severed. The solution to modern food and weight issues has little to do with eliminating carbs or fat, nutrient timing or anything else that keeps the mind focused on food. This is especially true for diets that emphasize what you can or cannot eat. In fact, this type of emphasis just reinforces the attention bias. You can't stop thinking about food, which is the very problem for people who have these issues.

Effective treatment means being able to understand your specific influences. True healing means learning and establishing new thought patterns that will naturally keep old ones in check. Only with these new, healthy cognitive associations will you be able to truly let go.

Behavioural tools—not diets—will eradicate indulgent food issues over time.

Chapter 3. Cues, Habits, and Your Emotions

We are all susceptible to unwanted thoughts or desires brought on by psychological or environmental cues. Not only that, we are also all just as vulnerable to attaching emotions to such cues.

To recap, a cue is a sight, smell, sound, thought or feeling that triggers and captures your attention, and can stimulate you without your conscious awareness. Moreover they may exist in combinations, compounding their influence. How susceptible you are to any given cue may be determined by its intensity or frequency, along with your own predisposition to be vulnerable to it. For some people this can play out as full-blown diet and food issues, while for others food is no issue at all. That said, this is determined by psychological and environmental influences, and it has little to do with metabolism.

Environmental cues are pervasive and complex, yet also hard to observe, because what triggers one person may not influence another. It depends on whether some kind of psychological connection has been made or not. Once a connection is made between emotional reward and an indulgent food cue, these cues will direct our attention toward them.

This is neurally wired into our brains, and is an understandable response. It is not a character flaw to be suffering any food, diet, or weight issues in our modern age. It is more accurate to say that these issues are psychological and biological challenges.

Most people who suffer from indulgent food or diet issues, and who are prone to the influence of cues have one thing in common. Namely, they are aware of the undesired thoughts, but they're not aware of what *drives* them. And it's only once this is decoded that the issue can be remedied.

Think of your favourite song—the way it can transport you to a past experience so real that it could bring your tears. Or a certain fragrance—the beach, nutmeg or a new car for example. Food cues do the same thing. The reverse is also true. A memory can remind you of a song, a time of year, or any number of things.

Food cues and memories, have a mutually reinforcing influence that has nothing to do with knowing whether a certain food is good for you. Cognitive association and emotional reward always trumps rational thought. This is yet another reason why adhering to a strict diet never lasts, and now that you know, you don't have to feel guilty about succumbing to a food indulgence.

* * *

We know, based on the biology of weight control and the brain's survival instincts, that when the brain or body effectively perceives a risk of food deprivation—as in extreme dieting or contest-dieting—it will increase its drive for food reward. When calorie levels are too low for sustained periods, the drive for sustenance increases, but so does the rewarding experience of eating. You are more driven to get food, and the reward is greater when you finally eat. On a diet, food is the absent reward, and in a calorie-deprived state humans are wired, physiologically *and emotionally* to pursue that reward.

Scientists have repeatedly proven that exposure to indulgent and rewarding food experiences followed by deprivation create the strongest sensitizing effects. If you have ever been on a strict diet, you know that over time the idea of an indulgent food reward takes on greater mental and emotional power within your mind. You become consumed with thoughts of your favorite foods. This has to do with the neurotransmitter dopamine. The cycle of deprivation, indulgence, further deprivation and so on illustrates how all overly restrictive diets fail us. The act of starving yourself only guarantees a ravenous appetite. So, for every strict diet, there is an equal and opposite binge period, as many people reading this I'm sure have experienced.

H.U.N.G.E.R.

I have adapted the acronym H.U.N.G.E.R. to stand for "How Urges Neurally Generate Emotional Response." It is a self-reinforcing cycle.

Here's how it works:

A cue triggers a dopamine-spiked plea for your mental attention. The dopamine surge causes an attention-bias to pursue the reward, in this case a food indulgence. The actual emotionally rewarding food experience from the indulgence leads to opioid release. This in turn creates a cycle, producing dopamine and opioids that together stimulate further future indulgences. Over the long term, the cycle gets heightened and intensified.

Another phrase used to describe this cycle is **"cue-induced anticipation."**

This phrase speaks to the well-documented association between various environmental stimuli and emotional cues to pursue a certain line of behaviour. Reactive, impulsive eating is often the natural result of a cycle that began originally with food deprivation or denial, which engenders a level of preoccupation with food or food issues.

Once this cycle is set in motion willpower and resistance only go so far. The more time and energy that's spent resisting cues, the more power they'll have. Eventually you'll give and satisfy your perceived need—maybe not immediately, but soon enough. Anyone who has blown a diet knows this is true. I like to use this phrase:

"What you focus on expands."

Once you create an emotional struggle with an associated psychological food cue, the only way to relieve that struggle is to give in to it. But then the cycle begins again. This is part of an inherited psychological drive for survival.

Again, it is not a character flaw. It is biology.

Conditioned stimulus-responses occur much quicker than people realize. In one study test subjects were given a high sugar, high-fat snack for five consecutive mornings. For several days afterward, the subjects craved something sweet at the same time each morning. I use this example to show just how quickly a conditioning stimulus can lead to a cognitive association. Habits are so easy to form concerning food, and so difficult to break when food as a rewarding emotional experience is reinforced.

How These Habits Are Created in Physique Competitors

Coax the body and it responds. Force the body and it REACTS.

I have worked with physique athletes for decades. Many of the competitors I've coached come to me with diet-induced eating disorders and food issues that they never had prior to contest dieting.

The strict contest diet eliminates not only food quantity but food *variety* as well. Beyond that, while in this state of caloric deprivation and restriction, competitors also overwhelm their bodies with the rigorous physical training.

Over time the physical state of hunger and the emotional state of exhaustion create a heightened state of arousal regarding food as an emotional reward. As the contest draws near, the cognitive association between the food reward and the post-contest celebration swells. The emotional impact and anticipation consume the competitor's every waking thought, and instead of looking forward to their time onstage to showcase all their hard work, they only look forward to eating. For weeks this attention-bias toward food indulgence has flourished. Once the reward finally comes, the cycle of arousal-urge-response is set in motion. This experience regularly leads to full blown weight problems and eating disorders. And fitness competitors are supposed to signify the pinnacle of health.

The competitor gains bodyfat after the competition, so they believe the solution is another competition to get back in shape. Only now they're just repeating and reinforcing the weight loss/weight gain cycle, and digging themselves in deeper.

A mindset of food deprivation "sensitizes the neural circuitry of the brain that mediates reward-seeking behaviour." (Carr)

Remember, habit means that "cognitive effort is surrendered to automatic response." This is not inherited laziness. It is a repeated cycle that is better explained as "earned and learned." Only acting with awareness can a cue, reward or habit cycle be replaced. This is neural, not simply behavioural. Behaviour is just the learned response and the end result.

Looking Toward a Solution: Part I

To live in this era is to equate certain foods with reward. Maybe as a child when you were sad, you were given a treat. If this became a pattern, the emotional desire leads to the behaviour of eating. Except now, because a pattern has formed there is an emotional 'learned association' between that particular emotion and indulgent eating behaviour. Over time we may lose a taste for the item, but it still unconsciously represents reward. There are people who recall eating a whole bag of chips without remembering its taste, or enjoying it. Yet they also admit to a lack of control in their ability to close the bag before it's been emptied. It is not the taste of the food indulgence that is delivering the reward but the relief.

This is how diet, food, or eating issues can play out for millions of people. Anxiety seeks relief. Diet, food, or eating issues become sources of relief that only propel a fresh wave of emotional tension and anxiety.

Begin to question the underlying sources of your anxiety. Instead of berating yourself for eating an entire bag of potato chips investigate the thoughts you had prior to tearing the bag open. How did those thoughts make you feel? You already know what action the feelings led to. Over time, working backwards from the undesirable food-indulgence behaviours, you will gain an awareness that will loosen the grip of your unconscious mind.

Further knowledge of nutrient components and concepts might seem like a way out, but ultimately they will not change or alter a cue-habit-reward cycle, not any more than me gathering a knowledge of the internal combustion engine will help me parallel park a car.

The key to eradicating eating, diet and food issues is cognitive learning.

Recognizing your specific cues will help to set you free. At first, even once you become aware of your cues, you may experience anxiety. This stress could initiate the negative food-indulgence spiral. I urge you to be patient with yourself.

Chapter 4.
Neural Circuitry in the Brain

A massive amount of research has been conducted on cue-induced anticipation and reward-seeking behaviour. Until recently, the focus was on drug and alcohol addiction, but over time, as more research has been done in related fields, it's become obvious that the findings are just as relevant to the modern food and diet dilemmas suffered by so many people.

The Opioid Center

The opioid circuitry of the brain is the pleasure and reward center we have been discussing. Stimulating the opioid center of the brain with indulgent food intensifies the craving and eventually the urge for you to "score" more. Just like drug abuse, the longer and more often indulgent foods are "used," the more intensely the opioid circuitry is activated.

This works in much the same way as exercise-induced endorphins, however the taste-pleasure-opioid response is stronger—more in line with drugs like cocaine or heroin. The result of consumption, whether it's indulgent foods or hard drugs, is an experience of reward and pleasure. This is why I have been saying for years that sugar has a narcotic effect.

Indulgent foods relieve tension, thereby providing comfort, acting as prescription or recreational drugs. It gives a whole new meaning to the term "comfort food."

Dopamine

The neurotransmitter dopamine motivates people's behaviour and compels them toward appealing food. More importantly, dopamine is directly connected to another survival response known as "attention bias."

For our ancestors, being both prey and predator meant having to develop keen "attention" to the prevalence of either food, or being pursued *as* food. The attention bias (or the potential for it) is directly wired into our neural drive.

Attention bias is defined as "the exaggerated amount of attention that is paid to highly rewarding stimuli at the expense of other (neural) stimuli" (Kessler 41). This is non-metabolic. But this attention bias can give indulgent foods a very prominent place in someone's mind, especially in our modern era. This is especially true if this begins in childhood.

Attention bias means that the more indulgent the food is, the greater the attention it will demand from people susceptible to that specific influence, and the more often and intensely they will focus on it. As an element of attention bias in terms of the reward cycle, this means they are most likely to work to pursue this focus of their attention bias.

Now, although this part of the cycle is non-metabolic, it can certainly be tied into the drive of actual physical hunger. Studies show that very hungry animals get frenzied and hyperactive just before they know they will be fed. Just like I've witnessed with my own dog, I have seen the same thing with extreme dieters and physique competitors. People who attain unnaturally low levels of body fat will have that condition be accompanied by intense hunger levels, and this skews their attention bias toward food.

When an extreme dieter or contest dieter is in this condition, and they know they will get a cheat day or cheat meal in the near future, they often cannot sleep for days beforehand. This represents the strength of the attention bias in the dopamine reward cycle.

For sure, physical hunger can certainly influence the attention bias toward indulgent foods. This becomes just another reason why diets fail over time. But at the end of the day, this is not a metabolic or nutritional issue, even if it affects metabolism and hunger. It is still a cognitive awareness and psychological issue.

Dopamine plays a role not only in the search of food, but in the search for love as well. It is the dopamine influence that stimulates and sustains the bonding in many animal species. Dopamine's role in creating perceived emotional value and connection to a reward stimulus is incredibly strong. This role of dopamine in search of love in animals has led to some interesting conjecture among diet specialists in psychology as well.

For some people this whole opioid cycle in connection to food could serve as a form of self-nurturing, not just hedonistic self-indulgence. There have been many research findings that show a tendency towards being overweight, or a tendency towards food issues, for children growing up with an absent parent, or without emotionally nurturing parents. In these examples, food becomes an emotional surrogate, and the value of comfort, love, and security provided by food is a powerful force. We now know that this dilemma is not solved with external solutions like diets but with cognitive awareness. Only then can we respond in healthier ways, and thereby replace these food cues and their emotional rewards.

What these disorders share in common is a high degree of sensitivity to sensory stimuli (in this case food) combined with a perceived loss of control and an inability to feel satisfied. These emotional connections are usually also combined with obsessive thinking.

"Priming"

We have all heard the expression of being "primed" for something. Priming is another of the signals to the brain given to us by evolution. Priming works by triggering pleasurable memories and lighting up the brain's reward circuitry. For some people, just *thinking* about indulgent foods will produce this response.

This concept of priming is something the food industry actively and successfully capitalizes on.

When an AA member warns, "one drink leads to one drunk," that's priming they're talking about.

For some people, a single dose sets up a primed response to pursue more. I have witnessed this in my practice my entire career. If a dieter has gone a long time without the stimulus of an indulgent food, and then has even a tiny little bit it as a reward, priming kicks in. Often a binge occurs (especially in inexperienced physique-competitors post-contest).

A sip of wine, a nibble of chocolate, ice-cream or whatever can trigger the priming response and annhialate any carefully wrought mental restraints that were previously in place.

Emotional drives trump rational thought.

Make no mistake here: when someone is hungry, or super hungry from extremely restrictive dieting, then almost any food at all that is perceived as emotionally rewarding will have a priming effect. Any good dietician will point this out as a risk to dieting in general.

At this point, having a little is usually *impossible.*

Foods that Trigger the Priming Effect

Would you lose control eating brocolli, apples or carrots?

What about pizza, candy or chocolate-chip cheesecake?

The more indulgent a food is, the greater the impact and intensity will be of its priming effect. And almost always these foods involve multi-sensory layering. It should not surprise you that combinations involving sugars, chocolate, or alcohol release the most dopamine.

Taste "has an acute emotional primacy." Because of this, emotional "reward value seems to be a fundamental dimension of gustatory sensation" (Anderson). Apples and carrots don't have multi-sensory layering, so they don't cause as pronounced a dopamine-release.

Variety

Studies on animals show that after eating a specific amount of one food, they tend to become satisfied or placated, and stop eating.

However, these same animals will *keep eating* if something *else* is presented to them that appeals to their taste centers. Despite being satisfied, they keep on eating, because hey, variety!

This speaks to the modern problem of having so much variety of food stimuli. In a single visit to a restaurant you can have appetizers, main courses, sides, desserts and drinks, all of which will ensure the repetition of the opioid/dopamine cycle. So many tastes and textures ensure that people eat *beyond* physical satisfaction and into the non-hunger-related reward value of the pleasures of taste combinations.

In nature, man had to eat food that was seasonal. There was no storage. Exotic foods were not exported. There were minimal taste sensations to ignite priming and the opioid cycle. Man, like the animals in the studies above, would eat what was available and be satisfied.

Moreover the taste-specific satiety engagement also explains why modern diets of single food emphasis will never work in our modern era of abundance. We have all heard of various single food isolated diets, like the grapefruit diet, the cabbage soup diet, the fruit diet, and now there is even the cookie diet and the ice cream diet. *None* of these will work because they run counter to the inherited neural networking aspects of our brains. We are omnivores. Trying to limit yourself to one or two foods will almost certainly ensure an unhappy binge-eating episode down the road.

What is important to note at this point is that the dopamine cycle illustrates the difference between goal-directed and habit-driven behaviours. There must be a cognitive and an awareness component beyond simple diet-behaviour in order to eradicate the modern diet dilemma.

Multisensory Input

When I say multi-sensory, I mean that food stimulation isn't just about our sense of taste, although it counts for so much. A one-year old baby with a small square of chocolate, for example, will almost always smile and giggle with joy as she smears it into her mouth. Why? Her brain's reward center has been engaged on a very basic level. This is especially true of babies because they have scant awareness or experience of other sensory and environmental stimuli connected to the reward experience.

As far as our other senses, fat, for instance, contributes to texture, like the creamy mouth-feel in a spoonful of full-fat ice cream. The sight of a thick, moist slice of chocolate layer cake can cause you to salivate, even if it's just a photograph in a magazine. Maybe you're salivating right now, visualizing it. Scent, as we all know, works magic on our appetites, and the sound of a steak sizzling and spitting on a grill entices us. For modern humans, the eating experience has travelled well beyond anything we engage in merely for survival. We even know what colors to paint restaurants in order to stoke our appetites, what music to play, and so on.

Then there's food engineering. Even something as simple a candy bar is a product specifically manufactured to produce a variety of specific sensations with each bite, such that the dopamine/reward cycle gets engaged.

As a child grows into an adult, the reward experience becomes more enhanced, because they'll come under the unconscious influence of additional environmental cues and other sensory stimuli connected to a pleasurable and rewarding food experience. If the taste and reward centers of our brain are part of its operating system, the external stimuli can be considered apps or software that engage our brain's functioning.

Multi-sensory food appeal goes beyond metabolism and even the biology of weight control. All the things we are taught as trainers—absorption, digestion, elimination and the nutritional composition of food—are a separate aspect of food and diet.

From packaging to its marketing to its appearance on your plate, there are multiple ways in which food appeals to us, and sometimes we can't tell which sensory inputs influence us the most. Some people are vulnerable to visual cues rooted in food presentation or larger portion sizes. Supersizing is visually and indulgently stimulating. Free refills of drinks or popcorn at the movies can be an added priming effect for people drawn to the value of "more."

But let's not forget the fact that taste by itself has a strong, emotionally rewarding connection to the brain, and this means you can't just simply ignore it.

Gordon Shepherd MD and PhD at Yale School of Medicine, said this:

> *"The industry is geared to over-stimulating the senses of the consumer so that they eat more. The goal is to activate the parts of the brain that are susceptible to being conditioned to finding a product desirable and then wanting more of it."*

When 1 + 1 = 3

Once you have "an experience" with an ice-cream sundae you anticipate the next sundae merely by thinking about it, and any of the environmental cues associated with it. The brand, a certain smell, or any specific association *makes* you think about it. This is part of your survival instinct for attention-bias in the dopamine cycle. However, even though one sensory stimulus, like taste, is enough to provoke the cycle in your brain, exposure to multiple stimuli will provoke a compounded amount of desire—much more than you would expect.

Taste plus smell are not a 1 + 1 equation in terms of stimulus response, but pack *three times* the power for stimulating the reward center. This is known as the "**superadditive**" effect of multi-sensory stimulation. Richard Foltin, Professor of Neurobiology in psychiatry, determined that fat and carbohydrate combinations of indulgent foods are the dietary equivalents of a speedball (a mixture of heroin and cocaine) for some people, and only for the taste-level of food experience. This drug-like intensity does not include additional sensory and environmental stimuli.

The same effects in the same centers in the brain.

More specifically, Foltin's point is that these drugs act on both the opioid and the dopamine systems, lending to far more intense enticements to repeat the behaviour. His theory is that indulgent foods work the same way once the "reward value" has been experienced and wired into the brain.

From my own professional experience anu observations, I must agree. I have seen very intelligent, strong-willed people, who still have food, eating, or diet issues, and this hypothesis explains their behaviour perfectly.

Remember that this is only the taste component of sensory stimuli. We still have to account for the countless variety of tastes and sensory inputs available that just a generation ago did not even exist. Moreover, it is not a coincidence that specific food combinations such as "sweet and salty" have emerged as the most popular ones in our current era of food abundance. These are the blends with the most power in the opioid reward center of the brain. The innumerable varieties of modern food creates a never ending capacity for desire and momentary fulfillment.

The more stimulating a food becomes, the harder it is to resist. What is stimulating to one person may not have the same priming effect on another, which is why it is so hard stop it with a "one-size-fits-all" approach.

Whole Food vs. Modern Food Products

The simplicity of whole food has given way to elaborately structured food products. These products are enhanced to be far more sensory loaded and rewarding than any food found in nature.

This is true of "healthy" nutrition bars, powders and processed organic items as well. They're all engineered to stimulate and reward your brain. The idea behind them is not rooted in longterm thinking but for immediate gratification. Foods like these are "healthy" only if you think about them in a vacuum. Sure, they include so many grams of protein and carbohydrates, and only so many (natural!) sugars, such and such vitamins and this much fibre—but they still have the same effect on your brain.

The more rewarding the indulgent food feels—even momentarily—the stronger the learned response cycle. This reward experience (the "feeling" if you will) is emotional, not just gustatory. This cycle of response creates automated behaviour, much like cigarette smoking.

So you can see the answers to questions like:

"Why do I keep doing this to myself?"

or

"Why do I keep blowing my diet when I've been doing so well?"

The key lies in the automated 'learned response.' In other words, if a habit can be learned, then it can be unlearned as well. But what this requires is *not* another diet.

Cognitive Restructuring

Often the advice to dieters regarding their reported

hunger is to "try not to think about it." (Um, what?)

Cognitive restructuring requires shifting the focus from undesired behaviours. Goal-driven actions like dieting or competing in a physique competition typically fail over the long term partly because the attention is directed at the very behaviours that trigger the problematic issues.

Active resistance is not a solution, and though it can seem counter-intuitive, it is often a part of the problem.

This is an awareness issue, not a willpower issue. The expression, "What you resist, persists," applies here. Trying to resist your desire and cravings for indulgent foods, or exposure to their cues, will only enhance your attention-bias toward them. Cognitive restructuring means finding healthier yet equally powerful mental and emotional responses to constant food cues.

Once again, when you fully understand the neural circuitry of the brain's reward center to seek survival and emotional rewards, it becomes easier to see how diets are part of the problem, and by themselves are never the solution.

Zebras and Pink Elephants

At some of my workshops we do the following exercise: I let everyone know that we have sixty seconds of quiet time, and for that minute, they are not allowed to move around, leave their seats or talk to anyone. Oh, and—they are NOT think about zebras for the entire sixty seconds. (Or pink elephants if you like.) Afterwards, I instruct them to write down how many times zebras popped into their minds.

Very few people succeed at this exercise. Telling someone not to think about something insures the presence of that very thing in their mind. Our minds aren't designed to not think about things.

That said, this exercise can become a powerful tool in terms of mental awareness if practiced regularly.

But food and hunger are different. As we discussed, once you have been exposed, as all of us have, to the reward value of food, it always has emotional priming value. Hunger itself is a physiological state. We are hardwired to pay attention to it, and telling people not to think about hunger is reckless. It will not work for long, and only instils the myth that diet is about willpower.

Moreover, there is nothing inherently *wrong* with thinking about indulgent food and its reward value, until and unless these are unwanted and undesired thoughts, preoccupations or obsessions. At that point, telling someone or even yourself to not think about food is even more ridiculous.

This is the emotional-mental connection in the triangle of awareness.

In the zebra exercise, tremendous mental energy is invested when making an effort to repress zebra thoughts. The mental energy is relieved by finally entertaining the subject that is creating the conflict. This is why people cannot follow the instructions for even one minute.

So when *food* is the issue—and we know food is not a neutral topic—it has even more power in the mind than something like zebras. Zebras are usually a neutral topic with no emotional connection or value. Yet telling you to NOT think about them, even for one uninterrupted minute, is not possible. So imagine thinking you should be able to suppress thoughts about food, especially when you are hungry from being on a diet, and when deep down you know the emotionally rewarding value that food has.

Research shows that trying to suppress thoughts like this is simply ineffective.

Trying to suppress this kind of thought or mental image is a lot like trying to hold a beach ball under water. Eventually it pops to the surface. When suppressed with force, it pops to the surface with even greater momentum. Trying to focus on not eating will propel you to eat, just like the beachball, regardless of your attempts to keep it submerged. It's a heck of a struggle, and it'll keep popping back up. Combine this with what we know about the emotionally stimulating effects of physiological hunger and that ball will surface with even greater urgency.

Shame and guilt are not empowering—they're destructive. Shame and guilt create self-fulfilling prophecies so that you end up binging or cheating because you're so afraid of binging and cheating and feeling guilty about it. It's backward, psychologically damaging and emotionally devastating. The whole cycle can start with one simple ill-advised diet and the unexamined mindset that drives it. The flip side is an eating disorder based on the denial of food along with an obsession with controlling foods. Anorexia is just as psychologically devastating and only makes things worse. Because now instead of trying to not think about food, you become obsessed with food—consumed with thoughts of food as your body wastes away from starvation.

No knowledge of diet and nutrition is ever going to help deal with these issues. In fact, a focus on diet and nutrition as a solution only worsens the problem because it reinforces the mindset to 'not think about zebras.'

Chapter 5.
The Emotions of Food

By now you have probably gained insight into your own personal relationship with food and weight. And of course you are learning how a deprivation diet can exacerbate any issues you face.

The individual perception of "loss of control" appears to be a growing trend even among those who are health- or body-conscious. For many of us, there is no longer a meaningful association between food and survival. In affluent society, food is now almost wholly a taste-experience, which invites even more emotional triggers and a perception of food-entitlement. Now, more than ever, emotional "cues," "triggers" and "priming" all drive indulgent eating behaviours and unwanted food issues.

Cues create desire. You drive by a Soft Serve on a hot summer day and your brain makes the connection that this food is "rewarding," regardless of any actual hunger. It is that simple. The cue creates the urge; the urge leads to the desire.

Your "cravings" are often this subconscious operation. People report to me all the time their cravings for this or that type of food. The food they crave is always something hyper sweet or fat (or both) not found in nature, like chocolate or peanut butter. The cravings are often reported *as* physical hunger, but what they really represent are emotional urges *interpreted* as food cravings, when in fact it they are emotional cravings. What, exactly is craved, is "a form of self-indulgence," which I will get to.

The Power of Memory and Cues

The ability to learn and store information regarding rewarding food experiences is to sensitize us for future cues that will bear the fruit of another emotionally valued experience. The cues will in turn bring up memories.

Memories themselves can drive arousal. According to Kessler, once that happens, "we repeat the actions that lead to the pleasure" (139). More importantly, "the more multisensory the stimuli, the greater the reward and the stronger will be the emotional reaction, and therefore the more potent the memory-influence. And the more potent the memory, the more powerful are the cues again" (139).

The more habituated a behaviour becomes, the less aware we become of its initial emotional drive. For instance you may initiate a habit of eating during times of stress. Eventually you eat *because* you are stressed. You now are influenced by the memory of something pleasurable occurring simultaneously with something stressful and the subsequent temporary relief you felt. As the behaviour becomes internalized, less stress is required to drive the behavioural response, and an automatic habit is formed.

The Paradox of Emotional Reward

Some experts believe that food does not relieve stress or problems. They're wrong. The reality is that indulgent food issues *do* in fact deliver emotional relief from various unwanted mood states.

Food provides temporary relief, but it does not solve the problem, and in the long-term it may intensify the level of anguish.

Food here is an escape, a form of self-medication. But responding to emotional conflict or intense mood states with food only masks or relieves the symptom, and on a very short-term basis. It never travels to the heart of one's emotional turmoil. I witness this all the time in my practice, where emotional eating leads to a full-blown food obsession or eating disorder.

"It's not about what you are eating,

but more about what's eating you."

Emotional relief derived from food indulgence traps you in a cycle of unwanted behaviour. Over time you drift further away from the actual emotion that caused the unwanted behaviour in the first place. These avoidance behaviours take over to the point where they literally weigh you down.

The emotional conflict is merely *represented* by the food, eating, diet or weight issues, but it's the unsavory emotions and thoughts you must deal with in order to finally let go. No amount of food indulgence or distraction is going to truly satisfy the emotional drive behind it. Only once you can see the paradox for what it is can you do anything effective to stop it. Thinking that food is the issue leads to treating the symptom and not the cause.

Labeling, feeling, and no longer being intimidated, bullied or ruled by uncomfortable emotions are the first steps in ending your indulgent food issues. The food issues are ghosts. When you are ready and willing to face your emotions and emotional drives, you can then stop using food to make you feel better, worse, or nothing at all.

Over time, a specific stimulus-response disorder related to food can be demoralizing. When something as unimportant as indulgent food takes over your life, it can make you feel unworthy and weak. The resulting cascade of negative feelings associated with this trap of self-medication just makes it that much harder to solve the real problem. It becomes easier to just keep reinforcing it. It is quite a paradox.

Please know that stress does not only refer to a negative emotional state. It can be a level of intensity beyond which you are capable of responding to rationally. Upcoming nuptuals or travel abroad, an impending birth or a promotion at work are all examples of stress that can compel you to seek emotional relief from food. This too makes every indulgent food issue a unique one. As we struggle en masse, we suffer in our own ways.

Memory:
Emotional and Behavioural

Memory of pleasure or pain can lead to desire. Desire triggers and engages the cue-urge-reward cycle.

If this reward is denied, the desire for it increases. At this point, a "willpower" commitment to a diet (for example, thinking, "I can never eat X foods again") will almost certainly intensify your desire for "forbidden" foods.

It is a memory connection that is engaged here, not any kind of metabolic profile. Since each memory-associated food reward is individual and dependent on your specific memories and associations, it makes zero sense to assign a generic, one-size-fits-all diet to any client seeking a weight-loss plan.

I like to use the example of Grandma's sweet potato pie. The pie is associated with joyful, loving family memories and celebration. It calls to mind feelings of being cared for and nurtured. The pie itself is a strong

nal memory cue, and conversely, the affectionate emotions are a cue for the pie.

I myself never had grandparents around, let alone a grandmother who cooked or took care of me. But I know someone somewhere did, and that this scenario is true for them.

Then there are "play-lands" located in popular fast food chains that combine food with fun and family bonding experiences. These color-saturated zones provoke strong recall associations in the brain. (Those fast food places know exactly what they're doing, by the way.) This strategy of "food stamping" can be as simple as putting a prize in the bottom of a cereal box. Food then becomes hot-wired to compel us to think about, respond to, and most importantly to 'feel' that triggered desire again and again.

Emotional Expectancy

There are **two major ways** that emotion operates with respect to food:

- When you expect the indulgent food to bring pleasure (as in say, a post-contest diet anticipated meal) the expectation itself amplifies the emotional reward value. This is **positive** reinforcement.
- Conversely when you expect food to bring *relief* from distress this also intensifies the perceived reward value. This is **negative** reinforcement.

In the post-contest period, competitors often experience disproportionate amounts of stress that cry for immediate release. Since eating is now the chosen behaviour associated with intense emotions, eating is what happens, even though ironically, stress about eating is the source of the stress. If one diet attempt leads to another the intense focus on food can become a debilitating obsession, either through obsessive denial, or through cycles of indulgence and restriction. For sensitive individuals, the cycle can last years. I witness this over and over in my practice.

The reward value in the example above is emotional expectation, regardless of positive or negative reinforcement. The eating of indulgent food occurs because of the the expected reward, not because of the actual enjoyment of the food itself. Many of my clients who experience social anxiety carry chocolate with them for potential uncomfortable situations, because they've learned to expect relief by indulging in a rewarding food indulgence. It is not so much the taste of the chocolate that is craved, but rather the feeling they expect it to give them.

The only way to stop the aroused emotional state is to eat the desired food. But this is a form of self-medication. In this sense, food is not the problem. The heightened arousal is the problem. (By the way, I find this diet-induced heightened state of arousal particularly prevalent in low-carb dieters.)

This is natural: starving for extended periods is unbearable. Tempers flare. Irritability and agitation deface the most innocuous exchanges. Anyone who has been around an extreme dieter can attest to this. It is not unusual post-contest for competitors to suffer anxiety, sadness and emotional emptiness (dysophoria). These very states lead to a heightened arousal. At this level, merely *thinking* about food can eclipse deeper painful emotions. *(Editor's note: Simply reading this book can find you face to face with the bottom of an ice cream container. Do not be alarmed.)*

To control your eating you have to learn to **control the heightened state of emotions.** It is *not* the other way around, as the diet industry would have us believe.

The anticipation of feeling better—even in what is ultimately an act of self-sabotage—puts people in the state of arousal that once imprinted, is no longer a pursuit of relief anymore, but a state of wanting in general.

Thomas Wadden put it this way: "food can be used to relieve an aversive emotional state, whether it is boredom, mild dysphoria, or more intense distress. A lot has been written about using food to escape awareness; that you are really trying to get away from yourself, get away from the negative or stressful mood that you are experiencing. A lot of this is mood regulation by food" (qtd. in Kessler 284)

Childhood: Then and Now

Not only is there far more emotional stimuli for food surrounding children these days, there is far less impetus to exercise.

Barry Levin of New Jersey Medical School, conducted a study on rats that gives us great insight into how easily weight issues can begin in childhood.

For the experiment, he bred one strain of rats to overfeed when a high calorie diet was available. (This sounds familiar compared to my own childhood!) The overfeeding produced an obesity-prone rat. The other strain of rat he studied was bred to not ordinarily overfeed. He called this group the obesity-resistant rats. These rats typically curtailed consumption after a period of overeating, much more than the obesity-prone rats.

This speaks directly to the prevalence of food in the reward cycle of the brain. Anything that promotes overeating, like a diet, can lead to constant over-feeding without restraint. Indulgence in palatable, convenient foods without restriction is a good predictor of obesity as time goes on.

This often begins in childhood, and children are frequently exposed to modern convenience and hyper-palatable foods without education or parental guidance.

Research have shown that overweight children fail to regulate their food intake when they are confronted with temptations such as the intense smell and taste of appetizing and indulgent foods—just like the obesity-prone rats. The children's sense of "enough" has been disrupted, simply by their environment. In overweight children, like the obesity-prone rats, this is all a matter of the cue-arousal-reward cycle.

If children are allowed unlimited access to indulgent

foods they will tend to eat them without restraint, because restraint is an adapted and learned skill. This research gives us clues as to how indulgent food, diet, and eating issues can manifest very early on, and also how and why they may be different for each individual.

It is not as easy as simply addressing general diet habits; you need to address how and why and when and where these diets habits formed. Childhood gives enormous clues as to the potential for future weight, diet, eating and food issues.

For instance (and this is just a hypothetical example) let's say a child is an only child. He comes home from school and his parents work. He has no siblings for interaction. And if his home is fully supplied with easy to prepare, no clean-up-required foods, then, since he's a child, he will likely indulge in them.

When these foods are processed, highly refined combinations of sugar, fat, and salt, they can have tremendous power in terms of creating and enforcing the psychological cycle of food as an emotional reward.

As the hours and days accumulate, food may become something more for the child—an emotional distraction, or a means of self-nurturing or a reprieve from boredom.

For a young mind without structured meal times, as the study shows, it is understandable that self-regulation might very well be improbable or impossible. When food is coupled with other mindless activities, like video games, television, social media, and so on, then even less attention is being paid to food regulation.

Food Hedonism

Hedonism is defined as seeking pleasure in the form of complete self-indulgence.

In psychology, hedonics deals with pleasant and unpleasant feelings. The food industry looks to five hedonic factors:

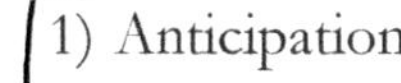

1) Anticipation

2) Visual appeal
3) Aroma
4) Taste and flavor
5) Texture and mouth-feel.

This is some of the most vital information the food industry utilizes to guarantee its vast influence and power over our tastes and appetites.

In the modern era, people feel entitled to eat what they want, when they want, and often as much as they want. The food industry makes sure they are bombarded by stimuli that reinforce this attitude. The irony is that the diet and fitness industries combat our sense of entitlement by promoting ideas about permitted vs. forbidden foods, strict diet-rules and so forth.

Modern diet corporations like Jenny Craig, NutriSystem and Weight Watchers persuade people to purchase "their company's" special diet with an attached indulgent-value: *"You can eat lasagne and indulge in your favourite desserts... if you do it OUR way."* This type of marketing is a direct appeal to food's hedonistic value, especially overweight people. Unfortunately it is a lie.

Food hedonism is different from self-medicating. I've had overweight people tell me with indignation, "I should be allowed to go out for dinner occasionally and enjoy myself." The subtext here is a fantasy of indulgence without consequence. It's infantile narcissism. These people tend to snack frequently, and scoff at its effect on their weight.

The hedonistic eater believes they "deserve" their food reward. They defend their indulgences with self-righteousness, which, frustrating though it might be, is understandable given the fast-paced, have-it-all nature of modern Western society. Food preparation takes time from our busy work schedules, doctor's appointments, personal training sessions; eats into time with our children and their myriad after-school activities. Perceiving food almost as a mini-vacation can lead people to perceive an eating experience as an entitlement.

Do any of the following "reasons" for indulging sound familiar?

I have PMS.

I just ran three miles.

I've had a really stressful day.

And so it goes. You could probably make your own

list. It might make you laugh out loud.

Food hedonists are hyper-involved in the act of eating and enjoying, but disconnected from the physical or emotional consequences. Additionally, this is not a shared experience, but a private self-pleasuring one.

The Psychological Negotiating of the Food Hedonist

Psychological negotiating is a tactic used by food hedonists to justify overeating, indulgent eating or mindless snacking. Eventually even small disruptions warrant rationalization and subsequent indulgence. The danger here is that in defending sabotaging behaviours, food hedonists are often primed to deny any responsibility for their weight gain.

Disinhibition of Eating

One of the more damaging behavioural effects of any emotional eating problems can be labelled as **"disinhibition of eating."** If someone blows her diet just a little, and that transgression unleashes other restraints which throw off the whole day or even several days, that's disinhibition.

This is what happens for the majority of alcoholics and drug addicts. One bite is the gateway to a binge that only ends when the food is gone, even when the person is so full it makes them sick.

Many people coming off a diet go through these

periods, where disinhibition leads to binge eating. Then there are those who overeat at every mealtime. Still others may avoid social situations if copious food will be available.

Food avoidance seldom works. A vulnerable person might wind up in the social situation mentioned above and succeed at eschewing food, as the idea of gorging in a room full of people is mortifying enough to stop them. Still, the cue is set. Once they return home, or maybe even a day or so later, when they're alone, the disinhibition-response kicks in and they stuff themselves.

Looking Toward a Solution: Part II

Cultivating the ability to resist stimuli and food cues is futile. Stimuli and food cues will always surround us. What we must do instead is develop an ability to weaken their power. This is accomplished with enhanced mental awareness. Understanding the issues is the first priority, and the priority of this book.

People all over the world use food to celebrate, to bond with friends and family, and gain a sense of community. We can't avoid it, nor should we, and we certainly cannot pretend societally-driven eating situations away. Telling yourself you will never eat your favourite food ever again is unrealistic and punitive. Your brain is wired for it, and life would be bleak without indulging every once in a while.

The question is how to exert control in a healthy way.

And here it is:

The emotional reward of food must come from an emotional place of empowerment and choice, and never conflict.

To be conflicted about food, eating, and diet issues is to remain imprisoned by them. For some people this is their biggest obstacle. But with proper and healthy indulgence you experience the reward without guilt. You also acquire an attitude of utility toward food, minus the stronger emotional connections.

The reward value of food can never be quite shaken, so it needs the addition of wellness in some form. I advise many of my female clients to make the same emotional connection to food that they have with shoes. For women in particular (in a broad and sweeping generalization, I readily admit) food and shoes have much in common. Both can serve as an outlet for personal emotional expression that relieve stress or numbness without excess emotional baggage (as long as you're not overspending). It's about learning how, when and why to "eat the cookie or buy the shoes."

As much as I say this tongue-in-cheek, it is true. Many activities allow emotional expression and ease our tensions, without adding emotional conflict. The important thing is finding that healthy outlet for yourself. It could be journaling, golfing or shopping. Maybe it's getting a massage or laying on the beach with a trashy novel. The main point is that in order to let go of these issues, some other positive cognitive association *has to* be created. This does not mean swapping one problem or addiction for another. Mental awareness is at the heart of letting go of any and all food, eating, and diet issues.

Whether the issue is self-indulgence, destructive narcissism or self-medicating, understanding that these issues are all psychological is the first step to truly dealing with them.

Chapter 6.
The Food Industry vs. You

No, it is not some sort of conspiracy. It's just good old capitalism. Competition in the food industry is fierce and there are enormous profits to be made. The major players spend billions to zero in on what works and what does not. This includes everything from taste and texture engineering to marketing, to our most sensitive emotions.

Regarding the power of "habits" formed in the brain as automatic responses, this is especially relevant. One of the habits the food industry hopes you'll adopt is a sense of "entitlement" for indulgent food without consequence. Once this pervasive habit is formed, consumers then become emotionally attached.

The food and the diet industries are symbiotically intertwined, dependent on each other for profit. They're not against each other—they're in bed together. The marketing and advertising behind both industries goad us to desire indulgent foods *and* a slim waist line, like coaxing an unwitting animal into a steel trap.

What's really being sold to you?

Take a good look at the next few television food commercials you see. What are you really being sold? The answer is almost always "emotional play." The food industry knows that emotion will not be overridden by rational thought. The goal is for you make a subconscious, emotional connection toward a product that typically shouldn't have any power at all.

Food advertisements seldom tout quality or nutritional value, unless they are central to the emotional play. If the commercials do refer to these it is usually of secondary value to the images presented. Food commercials instead tout the taste, convenience, and reward-value of the food.

The goal is to get people to 'feel good' about the choice. This can be as simple as telling a mother that "Nutella" is part of a "complete breakfast," whether this is remotely true or not. The product is beside the point. The idea is that being a busy mother is nothing to feel guilty about, and easy to prepare meals that your kids will enjoy sells "good parenting" to the mothers, who demographically and statistically speaking (because the industries obsessively track the data) tend to be the shoppers in their households.

Effective marketing is itself a "driver"—an arousal stimulus if you will—for food indulgence and entitlement. Marketing reinforces both the emotional agreement and the emotional conflict of food as reward. This is so powerful in psychological terms. Just as with cigarette addiction, this constant bombardment makes changing unhealthy habits an arduous task.

***

Ingredient-wise, if a product has sugar as its most heavy component, then sugar must be listed first on the label, right? Of course. But if a food product uses several different kinds of sweeteners, those can be listed separately. There are over forty different types of sweeteners which may be as sweet as or sweeter than sugar. *But by adding these sweetening agents separately they can then appear further down the list on the food label.* This makes the food appear healthier. We see this tactic used all the time in children's cereals. Using several types of sugars and sweetening agents allows for these ingredients to appear further down the list on the label on the box. But what is the truth? The truth is the glycemic impact is just as great if not more than it would be using one type of sweetening agent. By reading the label the consumer or parent is swindled into thinking that the sugar load and impact is far less than it is in reality.

So while consumers think they are serving their best interests by reading the labels, they may not be getting the whole story. For instance the Frosted Flakes label says it contains eleven grams of sugar per serving. But that's a manipulation of serving sizes. Let me put it in perspective: if you were to separate the ingredients in the box, *fully one-third of the box is pure sugar.*

The way around this, as Michael Pollan suggests, is to eat whole foods whenever possible.

To simplify:

- Items with one ingredient are healthiest. (How many ingredients are in a potato? How much advertising is done for them? Will you ever see a potato commercial during the Super Bowl?)
- From there, eat foods with five ingredients or less.

Remember, indulgent foods are seldom healthy and more often than not are not what they appear to be. 'Nutrition' and protein bars fit this description. Do they fit the rules above? Are they one ingredient, or five ingredients or less? More often than not nutritional claims made by the food industry are nothing more than creative writing in action. This is especially true with niche markets like organics, supplements and the like.

Identity and Marketing

Another marketing tactic is to sell "identity." "Nature Valley" cereal-bar commercials, for example, sell an outdoorsy, adventurous experience in connection with their products. There is a specific demographic and "identity" to whom they are speaking: "Buy our product, and this will be you." The marketing is obviously deliberate. The commercial's success lies in its ability to cater to both your consciousness and subconscious.

There is a reason beer and Pepsi ads play at night during televised sports. To the food industry, "eatertainment" is tied directly to the emotional reward center of the brain. In the presence of the promise of reward, people suspend rational thought, and are drawn to the simple indulgent nature of the experience. The experience itself *then* becomes an emotional driver connected to the basketball game, the NASCAR race or the Super Bowl.

The food industry thrives on the fact that life, stress and any general unpleasantness we suffer are suspended during indulgent activity. Think of the cost of popcorn and soda at your local movie theatre. Crazy, right? And yet people (myself included) are willing to pay ridiculous amounts of money to "associate" a food indulgence with an evening of entertainment.

Coca-cola shells out millions to be the only "soft drink" at a sporting event. The money made at the actual event is not that large compared to what they're paid for exclusivity. But the value of emotionally connecting their product to the home team—to people's sense of identity—*that's* infinitely valuable.

Adult Baby Food

The production side of the game is equally strategized. There are no accidents in the modern food industry, from preparation to propagation. From McDonald's to McCormick's, the test kitchen plays a major part of bringing indulgent foods to market. This is known as "fingerprinting." Moreover, chemical flavourings, along with with sugars, salt and fat make certain foods taste like almost anything, and have addictive qualities. This is how we are "lucky" enough to have items like strawberry-watermelon bubble gum, candy corn flavored Oreos, key lime pie flavoured Greek yogurt, carrot cake M&Ms and hundreds of thousands more. (For more on the drug-like chemistry of food, see *Fast Food Nation*).

The food industry also, in the words of one expert, "create a mood of experience." And that mood of experience can range from the adrenaline rush of attending a sports event, to a calm dinner out to relax and unwind. Another industry insider said, "We transform technology into good taste—tastes to excite, tastes to stimulate, tastes to comfort, and tastes to linger." (qtd. in Kessler p. 118) The word "*linger*" indicates the industry's aim for people to choose their product again and again.

When layer upon layer of complexity—including texture enhancements—is built into food, the stimulating effects (remember our friend dopamine) become more powerful. The industry counts on this. Gaetano Di Chara, University of Caliigiari put it this way: "the complexity of the stimulus increases its association with reward."

Did you ever notice that indulgent foods require less chewing? This makes for more and faster eating. What started as a side effect of engineered texture enhancement ended as another coup for the food (and diet!) industry. Some people are also especially drawn to larger portions as well, as previously discussed. Once these oversized portions become the norm, satiety cues get disrupted.

The industry knows that overeating increases reward value. As John Haywood put it, processing food, or creating indulgent processed food, produces in a sense, "adult baby food." Creepy, right?

So, instead of eating slowly, with awareness, many people now gorge mindlessly, shovelling in more before swallowing the previous lump of goo. (If you desire comic proof, I invite you to watch people eat popcorn the next time you go to the movies.)

Once again, another simple unconscious mechanism that for thousands of years helped us regulate our bodyweights has been purposely removed from our eating-experience. Chewing initiates the digestive process. Not so with adult baby food. It's literally a recipe for overeating.

I often instruct my clients to make a meal from raw nuts (e.g. almonds), a large apple and a very large carrot. You'll also need a notebook, pen, watch or timer.

Here is the only rule: You must not take the next bite of any food until you chew and swallow the current bite.

- Write down the time or have a timer set and ready.
- Measure 20 grams of almonds. Eat one at a time. After finishing the almonds, proceed to the carrot. After the carrot, eat the apple.

- Write down how much time elapsed from the first bite to the last.
- Make an observation as to your current level of satiety.
- Add up the calories and write it down.

On a separate day but at the same meal time, repeat the experiment with a multi-textured food of equivalent calories—say a pizza pocket—and eat it as you typically would. After eating, compare the time it took to eat the pizza pocket to the time it took to eat the nuts, carrot and apple. After noting the time difference, assess your satiation and hunger. Did the pizza pocket satisfy your hunger? Did you want more?

Even if you already suspect certain results, I want you to try it anyway. The value of physically experiencing the exercise will impact you in ways you simply cannot predict or feel when only supposing the outcome.

This particular science is aptly labelled, "Sensory Science" or "Food Quality and Preference." Awards and scholarships are presented for innovations in this area. In his book, *The end of Overeating*, Kessler quotes Michelle Foley, a food scientist at Frito Lay. Speaking at the annual Pangborn Conference, Foley said that her goal is to make food "irresistible." Her "formula" for food pleasure is "sensory stimuli + caloric stimulation." (If you perform a search under "The Pangborn Conference" you'll find additional, enlightening research about food sensory science and enhancements.)

To make food irresistible, the goal is to enhance its sensory stimulating capacity, *as well as* its caloric impact in terms of mouth-feel, and more important "being" food satisfied. When you think about it, it makes perfect sense to reduce the chewing labour involved.

Exploiting the Food Industry for OUR Agenda

There's an industry report called "Profiting from Consumers' Desires for Healthy Indulgences" that sells in the food industry for $6,000. It outlines how to exploit consumer desire. Though I have no itention to buy it, I'm sure that I've outlined some of its content in these pages. We can use this information to mark a path toward *healthy* diet sustainability over the long-term. We can and must depart from the destructive mindset of short-term attention-bias, and indeed from food deprivation as a weight loss strategy.

So-called diet gurus, especially in the fitness industry, often prescribe plans that call for, 'no starchy carbs but all the fibrous veggies you want.' This may sound appealing at first, but regarding Foley's 'food-pleasure formula,' 'all the fibrous veggies you want' simply won't meet sensory and satiation requirements over time. Equally at fault is the common (among physique competitors and extreme dieters anyway), tilapia and green beans (or chicken breast and steamed brocolli) four times a day.

Another study called "The 'Crave-It' Study" (sponsored by McCormick's Foods) examines and capitalizes on heightened states of arousal that lead to the food reward experience. It yields some important information for the consumer, the dieter and anyone with food, diet or eating issues.

The study focuses on how people orchestrate their own manipulation, thereby provoking an indulgent food response. I find this fascinating. The results yielded three types of people, classified as:

1) The Classics

2) The Variety Seekers

3) The Imaginers

(They later added a fourth group labelled as 'People Seeking "good" Nutrition.')

People are studied as "types" to see what particular foods trigger their pursuit of reward. Then food items are created to cater to the type of person. It is not the other way around.

The bottom line is, multi-sensory indulgent food sells. The food industry knows it. Now we know it. Let's put it to good use. So while the food industry uses elaborate chemical and processing enhancements, we can learn the value of herbs and spices for producing a similar effect. We can layer natural, whole, multi-textured vegetables and other whole food ingredients to create dishes that satisfy, satiate and truly nourish ourselves.

Chapter 7.
Sugar, Salt, and Fat: The Ultimate Combination

I have a sweet tooth.

I was brought up with two older brothers and money was scarce. We used to heat milk on the stove, add strips of bread and brown sugar and go to town. Sometimes this was my dinner. Just writing the description makes me salivate. Of course none of us had any idea that we were inadvertently wiring the reward centers of our brains.

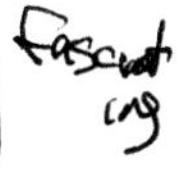

Cheap food tends to be highly-refined and layered with sugar, like the Frosted Flakes described previously. Sugar in all its forms has a direct effect on the dopamine response as we determined. It all seems innocent enough, but then the sensory science branch of the food industry emerged and now influences our food experience beyond our outsider awareness.

Traditional emphasis on food around the world used to focus on "satisfaction." The modern cultural environment has morphed to target food "stimulation." There is a big difference between the reward circuitry of modern humans in the current environment and how our distant ancestors related to their daily sustenance. This is the difference between modern desire, and ancestral need. More importantly "food satisfaction" now relates to food reward moreso than metabolic sustenance. This is a reality we cannot ever reverse.

I will always 'want' sweets. That is my food-connection and food-reward value. Early in life, eating the way I did, growing up in the environment I did, I wired my brain to be this way. As an adult this is my personal, specific diet dilemma. That said, I am fortunate to have been able to educate myself as to my own proclivities, and I have developed many ways to deal with my issue. But the sweet tooth remains.

The current food climate, if you will, exists in stark contrast to our unaltered biological drive for nourishment. Our brains evolved to survive in a food reality that no longer exists. Even during recent times—say the 1800s—there were no "supermarkets" nor any vehicles to get you to and from stores. But of course before that, you ate what you hunted and gathered. Can you imagine spending an entire day securing food for your family? The energy output versus the quantity acquired? Can you imagine a trip to the grocery store being frought with risk and no guarantee that you'll make it home alive, let alone with food for your family?

Developed countries—particularly North Americans—consume more of everything at a time when physical demands are less and less.

Think about this:

Early human diets contained about 10% fat.

Sugar intake was primarily in the form of seasonal fruit, when available.

There was no such thing as refining cane or beets or corn into sugar (there happened to be no diabetes either).

There were no refined meats, condiments or food storage.

Because of this, "natural" taste and food palatability were far more restricted. There would be far less emotional attachment to a food experience beyond survival needs, which meant biological and metabolic balance. Food would have little, if any emotional reward value. People's "tastes" were not nearly as developed, nor could they have been. This kept humans and nature in balance. In terms of the modern food experience this imbalance is also influenced by sugar, fat, salt. These refinements by themselves lead to an enhanced taste experience. And of course these enhancements fuel indulgence.

Ironically, it is unlikely people from a few hundred years ago would respond positively to modern tastes. The reverse is certainly true as well. But because of dopamine influences and such, the exaggerated stimulus of more sugar, more fat, and greater texture in food—all of these amp up modern man's pursuit of these various combinations and textures. (These are what Michael Pollan refers to as 'food-like substances.' Not quite food, but sure, food "like.")

And while this is "natural" in terms of modern pleasure pursuits, it has unnatural metabolic consequences. All indulgent foods can affect and stimulate the reward centre of the brain. Studies show that foods high in sugar, salt, and fat alter brain chemistry. (See the references section at the end of this book.) And then of course this circuitry becomes more pre-disposed and sensitive to repetition within the cue-reward cycle.

Before modern convenience, and before the layering of food with sugar, salt, fat and texture, man was not exposed to such cerebral influences: even though he was just as pre-disposed to it as we are. So while all of this certainly explains my "sweet tooth…"

…none of it explains what to *do* about it.

We'll get to that.

Sugar Brains

Culturally, apple pie has become associated with Thanksgiving, hot dogs with baseball games and so forth. All of this is because of our brain chemistry being altered by sugar, fat and salt, along or their endless possible combinations. We refer to these combinations as "texture layering."

Calorie for calorie, sugar in all its various forms has the most dominant influence in terms of altering brain chemistry. Moreover, rats will eat more when they are fed sucrose and corn oil, showing that the combination of fat and carbohydrate is more powerful than either component on its own. Add salt to the mix and arousal cues ignite even *before* the food is consumed. Aroma, texture and environmental stimuli add even more enticement, as you can imagine.

We already discussed a baby's first piece of chocolate and her subsequent joy. The stimulus-response effect is immediate. Furthermore, animal studies show that exposure to rewarding foods actually condition the animals to favor the *same place* where that food was originally consumed.

This means that environmentally, location can trigger the cue-reward cycle—the seashore, a neighbourhood restaurant, grocery store aisle—basically anywhere. Recall that when people were fed a sugary snack at a certain time of day, after only five days were besieged with "sugar cravings" at the same time in the same place. This is how potent sugar, and the texture-layering of sugar with fat, can be. If anyone experiences the intense craving for say, a margarita and a plate of nachos on Friday night around 5:30, well, you are not alone. *(Editor's note: True story.)*

There is also ample evidence that added sweetness and/or salt in the diet increases fat intake as well.

Let's examine this.

What do ketchup and mustard do for food? Ketchup adds sugar and salt, which enhances the sensory experience of, say that hot dog at the ball park. Mustard is usually added to a fatty food, like bratwurst, corned beef, etc. Why? Mustard also adds salt, which enhances the fat experience in the brain. Pickles, relish and Sriracha do the same thing, and all are likely to increase the amount of food and fat ingested.

Now think of condiments like "honey mustard." This is a multi-levelled, multi-layered flavour enhancement. that combines all three together: the triple threat of sugar, fat and salt. A trifecta of dopamine-stimulants in a single condiment. BOOM. The drug-like effects are powerful indeed. It is no accident that modern texture enhancements amplify the emotional reward value of a food experience.

Now let's take something as simple as a daily indulgence like coffee.

Coffee already includes stimulant value (i.e. caffeine). We all know that. For people who take cream and sugar, or even artificial sweetener and cream. This texture layering combined with caffeine enhances, via the stimulant value, the impacts of both sugar and fat in the reward center of the brain.

It doesn't matter if this registers in the conscious mind. Additionally, repeating the indulgence influences the reward values for both sweet and fat. This alone can cause cravings for either or both in *other* food experiences throughout the day, thus making dieting even more difficult. It can also pronounce the effects of enhanced texture of sweet and fat in a common daily indulgence. It works on a subtle level, but Simple daily indulgences like this just feed the reward cycle for seeking out multi-layered indulgent foods. This can make 'trying to diet' even more challenging.

(For more information, see Naleid, A.M., et al, "Deconstructing the Vanilla Milkshake" in the reference section.)

More Sugar, Salt and Fat

Starbucks attracts a younger and younger demographic. These consumers tend to look at coffee beverages as relatively harmless indulgences, especially when compared to known junk foods. But texture layering can be so refined that what seems innocuous on the surface is anything but. Recently at my local Starbucks, while waiting for my coffee, there was a group of young people in front of me. I asked one of them what she just ordered. She was happy to tell me she just ordered a S'mores Frappuccino, and to let me know how wonderful it was. It came to her as a 'drink' with a straw and whipped cream.

The young lady may have considered the calories (500 in a Grande made with whole milk!), the fat (20 grams!) or carbs (75 grams!), but certainly didn't bother to assess the Frappuccino's texture-layering impact and imprinting on her brain, which curiously, along with the ingredient list, is not handily accessible on the internet.

With all that we've covered (and uncovered) thus far however, we can readily conclude that the combinations textures in this drink are far beyond what anyone would guess. The added caffeine's stimulant value would almost certainly rewire her brain for irresistible future indulgences far beyond what any whole, unprocessed food would ever be capable of.

As if this weren't enough, because it is a drink, the Frappuccino gets absorbed far quicker than solid food. This increases its drug-like effect as well. It's the difference between a pill and an injection. Should this young lady enjoy Frappuccinos with regularity, it will reinforce her reward cycle for super stimulating multi-textured foods, and very well pave the way for weight, diet and food issues.

That's what I mean when I talk about the "modern diet dilemma."

The Bliss Point

The bliss point is the apex of gustatory pleasure.

The modern consumer has traveled light years beyond mere 'exposure' to multi-sensory food experiences. We now seek satisfaction in the farthest reaches of the comestible cosmos, and the food industry is more than happy to comply, as it formulates ever new creations for us to devour with abandon. A few recent fads come to mind—chocolate bacon, salted caramel, strawberry-balsamic, and one I found on the Disney food blog: a PB & J burger with bacon and jalapenos. Just. Wow. For a person from a mere generation ago, these types of food indulgences would annhialate the taste buds.

With modern convenience and multi-texture layering, the bliss point keeps ascending, and with it another of the natural, unconscious elements of weight control—unimpaired flavor boundaries.

I experienced something like this myself recently. My step-son is in his mid-twenties. He has no food or weight issues, and enjoys a wide variety of foods. The other week he bought some chocolate covered Jujubes, a treat he wanted to share with me on my cheat day. Interestingly, my step-son doesn't think of himself as having a sweet-tooth. He has no food-reward bias like I do.

But he loved those Jujubes. Meanwhile, I had one and didn’t like it at all. You would think that with my bias toward sweets, I'd love it. But it was far beyond my bliss-point, even as it hit a food-reward homerun with my step-son.

Section Two.
Solutions

Chapter 8. Introduction to "Solutions"

You now know some harsh truths when it comes to diets and dieting. It's disheartening to discover that your body is programmed not only to put on weight, but also to repel your attempts to lose it. This is the one-two punch of the physical side of the modern diet dilemma.

Previous means of unconscious, effortless weight control are no longer in place: gone are structured meal times, chew-labour, food preparation and daily physical labour. Additionally, snacking can and frequently does occur throughout the day and late into the night. Food storage and preservatives mean that no one has to depend on fresh seasonal fare to naturally limit their food choices.

This combination of factors multiplied by an endless array of strategically and chemically engineered offerings marketed and sold by the billion-dollar food industry unmoors us from what worked FOR our survival for over one hundred-thousand years until this very point in history—namely, our biology.

Regarding brain chemistry, you learned that sugar, salt and fat, along with their endless variations and combinations amplify and intensify the drug-like effects of food in the opioid and dopamine systems. Early childhood experiences with these flavor- and texture-enhanced products practically program you to repeatedly seek the reward inherent in these food products.

Only by restoring a food connection that utilizes our inherent biology and environment in ways that aid weight management and control can we ever transcend eating, diet, food and weight issues. But with all we now know about human evolution, biology, brain chemistry and the environment, how does one achieve such a seemingly insurmountable goal?

What does it take to change?

Overcoming diet and weight issues necessitates **becoming student of your own behaviour.** Awareness has everything to do with the mental, emotional and physical aspects of your behaviour and thoughts, and very little with the nutritional components of a 'diet'.

What is required to alter and change indulgent eating behaviours or food issues is, first, an opportunity to change them, and second, the sustained motivation to do so.

Consistently replenished mental and emotional resources are necessary tools that will help you locate and extinguish that learned connection to pursue reward via a food indulgence. I would suggest that you gather a support system as well—friends and family who truly love you and support your health and healing. So many people suffer from food-related issues in solitude and shame. They may fear seeking help or guidance, which is of course part of the problem.

If you feel guilt and shame about any of your food or eating issues, know this: hanging onto your painful feelings means hanging onto the problem.

A change-agent may be necessary to further the process—someone who knows the territory—a coach, friend or counsellor who works with you to help you identify and label your emotions; someone who can help you cultivate the motivation and tools to override, replace or disrupt your uninvited, unwanted thoughts, feelings and behaviours.

This is true of any kind of change-agent, whether it is to help someone overcome smoking, eating issues, substance abuse or physical abuse, for example. This is someone who understands behavioural impulses created by emotional drives in the cue-arousal-urge-habit-reward cycle—very well someone who has been there.

Going it alone or expecting immediate results indicate a lack of true commitment and undermine your ability to travel the healing path with self-love and kindness. Moreover, as typical daily stressors pile up, the motivation required to change habitual behaviours can wane. Stress wears down the will and the confidence to change. This is when your support system can buoy you most.

Solutions, Strategies and Tolerable Hunger

Real solutions lie beyond "willpower" or "trying." The change you seek does not come from any sort of twelve-week diet plan. A diet is simply another behavioural path to follow—a fallacy born of the fitness and diet industry. Your failure is the reason these industries earn billions of dollars. If their peddled solutions worked, the industries would cease to exist.

A "diet" is a Band-aid, not a cure. To conquer food issues you need strategies, and these must be holistic—mental, emotional, spiritual and physical.

Stress, anxiety, depression, shame and guilt leech your emotional strength and your capacity for self-restraint. Interestingly enough, on the biological side of the equation, food deprivation and extreme dieting almost always end up destroying the emotional capacity for self-restraint as well.

So the question is a matter of degree of hunger as well. Extreme, prolonged hunger might lead to weight loss initially, but it is damaging and unsustainable physiologically and chemically. That said, I'm going to tell you something that many people will find counter-intuitive, but is both mentally and biologically sound:

Make friends with a certain level of tolerable hunger.

In terms of cognitive awareness, you need to come to grips with a specific level of **tolerable hunger** as the *norm* for optimal function—mentally, physically and emotionally.

Food should become a means to satiate hunger, not "reward" it.

Understanding, working with and being able to "feel" true hunger and satiety requires a shift in perception. It is also a key component for overcoming any food, diet, eating, or weight issues. Real physical hunger requires that you make a distinction between want and need.

A bit of physical hunger means good things:

- It means fat burning.
- It means effective assimilation and digestion.
- It means an intact hunger-satiety reflex
- It means the end of confusion regarding 'being hungry.'

Hunger is Natural

Getting used to being mildly hungry is part of the solution to any indulgent food issue. People have been conditioned to think that they need to be "full" after eating. This is a very different mental construct than feeling satisfied.

Let me repeat: "being full" is not the same as "feeling satisfied." Eating for reward is much different than eating to satisfy hunger. Moreover, no amount of food will satisfy a hunger that is emotionally driven—at least not for very long. And then the cycle repeats itself.

How to become used to a certain level of tolerable hunger

- Choose smaller portion sizes and smaller meal sizes.
- Choose primarily whole foods, high fibre carbohydrates (including starchy carbohydrates), a little fat and a little protein at each meal.
- Eat several times a day.
- Ask yourself, "Is my hunger met for now?" Not, "Am I full?" It sounds easy enough, but many people do not seriously attend to this particular instruction. Asking yourself this question is a requirement.
- Know this: a constant state of tolerable physical hunger reflects the norm of our ancestors' experiences. Earlier humans had no weight issues—or deprivation issues—living this way.
- This connection needs to be a positive one. If the

idea of smaller portion sizes remains one of deprivation, you'll eventually rebound.

Anchors and Triggers

To develop emotional learning capacity, you need to clearly label your emotions in a relatable, resonant way.

One such example is the idea of "anchors and triggers."

Psychologically, these terms help you understand behaviour that draws you *toward* something you want (e.g. a balanced approach to food and eating), or pushes you *away* from something you don't want (e.g. emotional eating).

For instance, you are not going to be able to stop an anchored habit like indulgent eating until you find a new emotional trigger to target and direct you toward the alternative.

Anchored behaviour is the reliance on various stimuli we've come to depend on for comfort or familiarity. It doesn't matter to our brains if this behaviour is self-destructive; once it becomes anchored and habitual it's it's up to us to deal with it.

Negative, unwanted behaviours, at some point become **habits** as a result of certain stimuli strongly connecting to a sense of emotional reward. If you want to fix things, **replace** the unwanted food-indulgent behaviours with *pleasing* alternative behaviours (i.e., alternative triggers) that have nothing to do with food, and contain an equal or greater emotional reward value than the current anchor provides. Know that there are far more important things to occupy your mind with than thoughts of food.

The driving force behind this is the idea is that the anchored behaviour is a food issue that is no longer desired on a conscious level. This is important to acknowledge because it has value in terms of self-motivation.

Selective Memory

What is selective memory? And why can it cause such destructive behaviours?

With selective memory the "selective" element is the positive aspect of the behavioural-indulgence. Your mind selectively pays attention to the emotional *reward* of the behaviour or thought—even if that behaviour or thought is self-destructive in many other ways. The negative or neutral elements involved are "selectively" left out. This is what can give "anchored" and habitual behaviours such power.

Self-restraint dissolves under the influence of an emotional trigger. It doesn't matter that you'll later regret. That's not how the brain works. Ever reached for the peanut butter jar, when you "know" it's a destructive habit that you always come to regret? How about that third glass of wine when you know that two is your limit?

Well, selective memory is why, in that moment, you reach for it *anyway*. It's not until afterwards that you remember all the reasons you are better off saying no. This is also why such habits can be so difficult to break. Willpower cannot stand up to the power of selective memory.

The reason diet setbacks are so common is because the neural connection to the reward is so strong. When presented with an emotional conflict or uncomfortable situation, your brain relapses to the unwanted behaviour. Selectively you believe the wine, or the peanut butter is going to make things better.

Self-restraint is a cognitive skill. The loss of self-restraint, because of inner emotional conflict, is emotionally driven. And remember: in the moment, emotions trump logic.

These are disconnected elements of your triangle of awareness. The solution? They need to be reconnected. And only a trained mind and an *aware* mind will be able to harness and control its own emotional drive.

Awareness and Relapse

An aware, empowered mind can learn from relapse and weaken the intensity of future conflicts that typically trigger relapse behaviours.

This is why these labels for awareness are so important. It gives you a vocabulary and a structure with which to understand what's happening to you, both as it's happening, and afterward.

Setbacks, therefore need to be perceived as typical and

reasonable. Rather than beating yourself up for 'failing,' think of a relapse as an opportunity to grow and reinforce healthy, desired future behaviours. Overcoming food issues result from **a genuine feeling of emotional satisfaction or neutrality.** No one ever conquered their indulgent food issues through resentment, shame or guilt.

The ongoing sense that you're out of control is a lie that came to be accepted as truth. Low self-esteem is another falsehood that leads to self-sabotage, powerlessness or even apathy. The problem is the arousal cue for unwanted behaviour, and *that's* what we target. We're going to change it, both the behaviour's intensity and frequency. This will loosen the grip of self-loathing, if that's part of your experience.

This can only happen if an alternative can be considered at the very same time as an arousal cue. The only way to ever accomplish this is to recalibrate the current mindset. Your emotions do not control you unless you allow them to. Believing that your emotions control you is exactly what *allows* them to control you.

Learn to control your thoughts and emotions, and you eliminate any unwanted habit or behaviour. This is a skill that must be practiced until it becomes automatic and habitual. This is known as "habit reversal," and it is the topic of the next chapter.

Chapter 9. Reverse Your Unwanted Habits

Many of the strategies we are going to discuss will suit you. Others won't. One may work for one person, but make no sense to another. That does not make the strategy right or wrong; merely compatible or incompatible in its particular context. Also, and this is especially true for those suffering deeper issues, a combination of several strategies might work best.

There are no one-size-fits-all solutions. Although the strategies involved and their underlying principles can be outlined on a general level, the tactics employed will be unique to each individual.

FEAR

The most important element involved in habit-reversal is **emotional learning**. We addressed emotional learning in the previous chapter, but there is a level of responsibility here that bears repeating: you yourself need to be emotionally responsible; you need to be willing to learn, and willing to acknowledge, feel *and then dispense with* unwanted emotion.

Emotional avoidance (often "another diet") is part of the problem, and never part of the solution. In terms of risk-management, which we will get to, you need to adapt the acronym "**FEAR**" which stands for "**Face Everything and Respond**." Currently your unwanted habitual behaviours are "reactions" to stimuli. Using FEAR, you will learn how to "respond" to stimuli instead. This requires **impulse awareness.**

Any kind of positive change, in terms of behaviour, requires responsibility and **"response-ability."** This happens when you do the mental homework necessary.

Risk Management

It is unrealistic to think that any solution for indulgent food issues can occur without risk, stress or finding oneself in an environment rife with triggers. In terms of FEAR, risky environments and situations are the very opportunities that, when faced fully, allow for meaningful habit-reversal.

For example, avoiding social gatherings such as a

friend's birthday party or drinks with co-workers is risk management. The only way to eradicate these issues is to face the circumstances which trigger them. And until you hone a new **response-ability**, your unwanted habits are likely to continue. So the first thing to learn regarding FEAR is that risk avoidance only perpetuates your issues. And anyway, how long could you realistically live your life avoiding all social situations?

Over time, with full attention, you will develop a new level of awareness. Only by facing these scenarios can you break the connection between cue and emotional reward.

Part of risk management is knowing that if you cannot control yourself around a certain food, like sweets or peanut butter (two common possibilities) then you abstain from these foods while working on other awareness factors.

Risk management means facing environmental *cues*, not actual *foods*. Remember, an alcoholic knows he cannot have "one drink," but he may still attend his sister's wedding where champagne will be served.

Risk management necessitates the same kind of acknowledgement from you. If peanut butter is one of your reward foods, don't eat it. This does not mean "resisting" with the kind of mental anguish and conflict involved with "willpower."

Remember, the drink, the chocolate and the peanut butter are only the *behavioural outcomes* of something else. Risk management is all about exposing yourself to this "something else" in order for you to understand it more completely.

Cognitive Disruption

In order to achieve a certain degree of response-ability, you'll need to develop further elements of mental acuity, such as **cognitive disruption.**

What this means is *challenging the habitual sequence.* In terms of response-ability, something else must replace the steps that lie between the "cue" and the "reward." They can't simply be removed.

Cognitive disruption entails creating both competing thoughts and competing behaviours when you are confronting and recognizing cues of your unwanted habits. Competing thoughts must come before the competing behaviours, but the goal is to have both. The competing thoughts must be followed by a competing behaviour if you are ever going to eliminate your indulgent food issues.

The ability to create 'competing thoughts' must come from a place of personal empowerment—this is why emotional learning precedes an ability to create competing thoughts.

Competing thoughts must also be powerful enough to dilute the usual emotional reaction to a food cue or stimulus. This is what creates an initial cognitive disruption in the mind.

What Makes a Good Competing Thought

One way to accomplish this may be to think ahead to "outcome" without emotional attachment.

Here is an example of an *ineffective* competing thought:

> *"Well, yes, of course I want the ice cream, but it only makes my problem worse and makes it harder to resist next time. Therefore I should not eat it!"*

Perhaps you have tried this method to no avail.

So why doesn't the above competing thought work?

The problem is that this 'competing thought' doesn't really compete at all. It's logical, sure, but not strong enough to interrupt the cognitive sequence, especially when you're staring at the container of ice cream. All this, and you're still entertaining your initial desire.

Arguing with yourself over the outcome of acting on a behavioural impulse is really psychological negotiation under the guise of a competing thought.

Once you find a successful competing thought, you'll reinforce it and begin to break the cycle of cue/urge/habit/reward. Every little rupture in the cycle leads to a certain level of automatic cognitive disruption over time. This means that "abstaining" *in and of itself* may not be the best means to create habit-reversal, but it can play a role in personal empowerment toward cognitive disruption.

However, abstaining from an indulgent food cue is only one of a myriad of possibilities for creating and maintaining cognitive disruption.

Remember this sequence has to be something you can repeat until the initial habit is reversed or eliminated. Remember also the concepts outlined in earlier chapters: "thought determines behaviour" and, "thought determines the *quality* of behaviour." When you are exposed to food cues, which lead to unwanted habitual behaviours, you have options. Examine your thoughts for a range of possible mental images which can manifest a competing thought—one that will eventually lead to a competing behaviour, which is our ultimate goal.

Competing Thoughts:

Change the Channel

Think of your current unwanted thoughts and subsequent behaviours as one television channel.

Once a provocative food cue pops up on your TV screen, simply change the channel.

Mired in the reward cycle, it seems like you are stuck on one channel. But there are thousands of channels available to you in that very same moment. Pick up your remote!

** Click! **

Fully experience a cue that leads to an unwanted behaviour, and then challenge that cue with a competing thought. Remember, no negotiating, and no rationalizing. Don't argue with the current channel. Arguing with your television might feel vindicating at first, but if it goes on too long, you start to look like a lunatic, screaming at an inanimate object. The same is true of your thoughts. Are thoughts really much more than a television show playing in your mind?

This act alone, even before the behaviour is introduced, can help create enough momentum over time to break the cue/urge/habit/reward cycle. It's an excellent first step towards your desired habit-reversal.

Competing Behaviours

Most people fail because they just do not take the steps to go from competing thoughts to competing behaviours. They just do not see this new process through on a *regular basis.*

In order to have real impact over time, a competing behaviour should be planned, personal and proactive. Whenever possible these alternative choices should also be emotionally neutral. At the end of the day you are trying to unbind emotional reward from its resultant unwanted behaviour. This requires a good deal of effort and thought, because it entails a lot of "new" consideration. It also takes a lot of repetition of the sequence, if you are ever going to override the current habitual sequence.

One possible solution I have created to use a model for cognitive disruption is "Colour Therapy."

Colour Therapy as

Competing Thought AND Competing Behaviour

Colour therapy works at several different levels, all of which serve the goal of complete cognitive disruption-all the way from competing thoughts to competing alternative behaviours.

When confronted with a food cue or urge you need to call upon another image *immediately*. Immediacy is very important for creating competing thoughts. Color therapy serves this purpose.

The reason we use "colors" for creating competing thoughts and behaviour is because the mind can so easily call on any color, in a microsecond and without much effort.

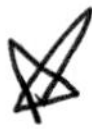

Here's how to use color therapy to introduce the competing thought:

- When confronted with an unwanted food cue or urge, immediately think of your favourite color. Never use black or white, and the brighter the better.
- Let's say I choose blue (you can change your color preference week to week, month to month, etc).
- Immediately after conjuring the color, spell it

slowly in your mind, then *see* the word in your mind: B-L-U-E.

- Now, imagine as many different types of blue as you can: Prussian blue, navy blue, royal blue, aquamarine, sky blue and so on. (Picture all the variations as vividly as you can before moving on to the next one. Take your time. Remember you are doing this during an undesired food urge.)
- Next, attach "blue" to as many things as you can think of in your head. So imagine blue running shoes, blue shorts, blue sky, blue water, blue jeans, and so on.

Already and with only a little effort, you have created a competing thought which disrupts that cue-habit-reward cycle. Remember that creating competing thoughts is only part of the process of habit-reversal. There must also be a competing *behaviour*. This exercise will help lead you there.

Now we use colour therapy for the competing behavior:

- If you are at home, imagine your drapes in dark or light blue, imagine if your sheets were blue, things like that. Look in your closet for blue clothing. Look for blue socks. Go get them if you have them.

- Go to your computer and do a search for "blue" and see what comes up, or maybe search for "blue shoes" or "bluest seas." See what images you can find.

The process must be practiced and repeated diligently and regularly. Your unwanted habit started a long time ago by making cognitive associations with food as reward. Cognitive disruption can and does lead to habit-reversal.

I like the color therapy approach: it is easy to do anywhere. It is personal; it is positive; it is practical; and it is empowering. It is also emotionally neutral, and anyone can do it. I recommend employing this strategy for an eight to twelve week period. It can be a powerful tactic to create enough cognitive disruption for full habit-reversal.

External Support and Habit Reversal

As previously mentioned, too many people try to fix their indulgent food issues on their own, and steeped in shame, guilt and silence.

Having someone else involved in terms of accountability and understanding can be a powerful *external* source of awareness in helping to overcome what is a powerful *internal* force. Coaching, not in terms of diet-adherence, but in terms of wellness-practice, is the best single tool a person can employ to accomplish habit-reversal and habit-elimination.

The problem lies within the arena of qualified coaching. Most 'coaches' qualified to help on this level are actually medical doctors, social workers, psychologists or psychiatrists, and that may be too big a step—financially and emotionally—for some people to take. I have not yet met a single coach in the fitness field who is even aware of this type of coaching, let alone who studies, researches and applies it.

If you do find a qualified coach, however, another benefit is the personal accountability factor. If the relationship is right, you are more likely to tell your coach something you cannot tell a friend or a significant other. This quality of intimacy without judgement often makes all the difference.

Moreover, most people with eating or food issues indulge in private. Being mature enough to be accountable to a coach can go a long way toward discouraging this type of behaviour. Once a behaviour is thwarted through any kind of cognitive disruption, such as the knowledge that your coach knows what you do when you're alone, the thoughts and emotions behind that behaviour can be weakened as well.

Think about it: not too many people binge in front of other people. This unconscious external constraint is a social restraint. It serves as unconscious "external" influence and accountability. But know that YOU are the one exercising that restraint. This goes back to the skill awareness, and as such, should be treated as a marker of imminent success.

What Successful Habit Reversal 'Feels' Like

To understand habit-reversal in neural terms, imagine brushing your teeth with your opposite arm, until it becomes 'easy' to do so. It's not necessarily natural or 'easier' than using the dominant arm, but it's still relatively easy. This is what habit-reversal 'feels' like.

This is in fact a matter of conditioning: the opposite hand can be used just as efficiently in place of the "conditioned" limb, with practice. Anyone who has ever had their dominant arm in a cast knows what this "re-learning sequence" is like. It's hard at first, but entirely possible.

Habit-reversal, in neural terms, "feels" the same way. You have already sensitized your dominant side for all these activities. Going back to them would be easy and feel right. The same kind of thing exists in your conditioned thoughts and behaviours that represent your food/eating/diet/weight issues. In neural terms, changing these sequences can feel awkward, and a little unnatural. But that is because of prior conditioning.

Chapter 10. Understanding Cognitive Awareness

It is amazing to witness in practice how many people will revert back to the willpower mindset during the reconditioning procress. The urge to resist temptation only ends up playing out the original emotional conflict. Worse yet, the phrase used in psychology that "what you fear, appears" or "what you fear, you energize" remains true as well. Willpower gives energy to exactly what you do not want, merely by focusing on trying to resist it.

The real battle is in learning to be smarter than your own original emotional conflict. Initially, a food, eating or weight issue is a simple equation: emotion drives behaviour.

Or:

Overpowering emotional impulse —> Mental fallibility —> Undesired behaviour or thought conflict.

As we have learned, this 'mindset equation' plays out unconsciously. The solution is to uncover and embrace and then reject the falsehood of this equation and adopt a **truthful one.**

That equation is: **intelligent awareness** *controls* **emotional cues that drive behaviour.**

Or:

Mental power —> Emotional input —> Behaviour —> Outcome—> Experience

There is an immense difference in thought, strategy and level of cognitive awareness between the two equations.

Understanding the second equation necessitates a shift in your own mindset. It is never a question of being 'strong enough,' as willpower supporters would have you believe. The first equation implicitly and falsely suggests this. Instead, it requires being 'smart enough' and 'aware enough' to deal with them. Cognitive awareness is a different kind of approach to eradicating these issues, and exists on a totally different level than willpower.

Whether you act out on food urges or not, being controlled by food mentally or behaviourally is to live in an emotional prison. Gaining conscious control over such issues stops the automatic cycle from engaging, beginning to end. The good news is that cognitive awareness can take place at any point along the cue-urge-reward process in order to interrupt its automatic response. Realizing that your food issues are a mind trap and a result of a single, narrow mode of thinking, leads you to entertain the myriad other possibilities. This is the beginning of the path to overcoming indulgent food issues.

This is cognitive awareness: the realization of your own possible 'choices.' You can select how to feel and how to think, what to feel. One method of 'choosing' is to look at diet as a 'lifestyle.'

Lifestyle is something you own, that never owns you. Drop the phrase, "I'm on a diet" and stop looking at diets as a set of rigid rules dictating permitted and forbidden foods. Rigid rules regarding "good foods" and "bad foods" is a form of diet-consciousness, which leads to diet-conscience—and in the end, to have a "conscience" about an "object" makes no sense.

You should start seeing diet as a thing you do or something you have; something you own. This lessens its emotional power. Your dining room table, bed or kitchen counter have no power over you. They are simply objects you own. What you objectify has no personal or emotional influence for you. If you have food issues, you just need to perceive your diet the same way.

Over time cognitive awareness and objectifying your perception of "diet" or "dieting" leads to removing its emotional impact from your mind. Diet just becomes something you choose to do. Over time, you learn to give diet the same level of emotional importance as say, washing your car.

Using the Engaging Mindset of Success

There are actually *unlimited* options for perceiving your indulgent food issues on a different plane of awareness.

An example is what I call "**the engaging mindset of success.**" Most people who succeed at anything in life engage the mind only in terms of succeeding at that quest, and nothing else. They remain detached emotionally, and do not entertain concepts such as 'winning or losing,' 'failure' or 'crucial".' The engaging mindset of success is mental empowerment. It sharpens cognitive awareness within the chosen field of concentration. Let's consider approaching a diet-mentality this way.

This is the difference between higher awareness, which employs emotions to think (creating passion and empowerment) and thinking impulsively with emotions which leads to reactions and unconscious levels of conflict and confusion.

Also, in terms of 'the engaging mindset of success,' it may help not only to objectify the concept of 'diet,' but to make it into a **game**. This can help remedy the faulty mindset of deprivation and denial, which are an attempt to remove the self from the diet equation—an attempt that will not work for long. Envisioning 'diet' as a game gives you a sense of control and participation. It is not difficult to do, once the concepts are explained and delineated.

What "Self-Restraint" Really Is

Self-restraint is not willpower; rather it is an immediate cognitive understanding of your unwanted desires. Behaviour follows either the unconscious unwanted impulse or the conscious immediate understanding of the impulse. We can also refer to this as 'purposeful self-restraint.'

Because your food-related issues are rooted in impulsivity in conjunction with a heightened state of arousal, being able to examine, label, and understand your impulses slows the impulse response, giving you the time to make a different, healthier choice. Once again, being able to do this is what cognitive awareness is.

Another characteristic to (re)acting on impulse is the perceived need for an immediate reward. This can also take place in the unconscious mind. Maybe you seek relief from stress and high pace, or maybe you seek relief from boredom. These can serve as emotional arousal cues to seek an emotional reward.

The cue to seek reward is always emotionally rooted, so to eradicate this you meet it with intellect—with calm, rational thought toward a longer term reward instead. While this can be akin to psychological negotiating, it can also be a step to impulse control—thereby enhancing your own cognitive awareness over time.

An Example

Say you have an arousal cue to go out for pizza and ice cream. At the same time in your personal life you have a goal to lose weight. The emotional "want" for pizza and ice-cream can be rationally negotiated, and you can think about how much you want to be in control of your eating behaviour. The rational mind negotiates with your emotional desire, and reminds you that you no longer want to keep suffering the negative consequences of a food indulgence. By reconciling your conflicting desires, using detached, rational thought, you supply objective intellect to the emotional field. This too, heightens awareness. It may not lead right away to impulse control and self-restraint, but it is a good beginning for getting there. **As long as this kind of psychological negotiation is not reduced to willpower or weight loss goals, it can serve a very positive purpose and release from a negative thought-behavior pattern.**

Self-Talk and Rationality

Self-talk serves as a wonderful tool for emotional awareness, if you follow through with it. Also, you must not meet emotion with emotion during self-talk, or you run the risk of agitating yourself further, because by bringing more emotion into the mix, you arm the issue, and disarm yourself.

The goal then, is to meet emotional want with mental clarity and rationality. This is the difference between willpower and cognitive awareness, as willpower only heightens the emotional intensity. Awareness dilutes it. The problem is that impulse-driven individuals lack what is known as response inhibition. They tend to react or overreact immediately, which prevents any level of awareness from developing.

Cognitive awareness brings rationality to the arousal impulse. Practice it regularly.

Name It and Claim It

Many people have lost their ability to properly label an emotion they are experiencing. The resultant confusion often plays out as emotional eating or food issues.

I had a client who was a confessed binge-eater, usually with chocolate or ice-cream. She could never figure out why this was the case and thought she understood her emotions so, "it couldn't be that." Then a personal issue arose. She related that she felt pain, embarrassment and anger. When I advised her to express her feelings in order to release them, she replied, "I can't do that. Right now I need to be supportive of the person involved." Instead of dealing with her emotions, she actively and consciously suppressed them, rationalizing that she was "being supportive." Her binge-eating continued.

An emotion cannot be released until it is felt and dealt with. Recognizing the immediate emotional triggers and arousal cues is a first step towards eliminating them.

Practicing the “name it and claim it” exercise keeps the mind engaged and invites more cognitive awareness.

If you cannot “name it, then claim it” then practice this sequence:

Practice the mental exercise to “*frame* it,” and then “name it and claim it.” If you feel this is you, mentally “frame” the situation around the emotion: where you were, what was happening, what was said and so on. Framing the incident is akin to creating a snap-shot. It is something you can look at from outside the situation, as an objective bystander.

Your Mental Strategy

Let’s see see if your attention and your intention are ‘compatible,' and if they’re working together. The key words here are “**attention**” and “**intention**.”

Regularly ask yourself, "What are my **intentions** with food or with my food issues?” Then within that observation ask the following: “What am I paying ‘**attention**’ to right now?”

The answers you discover will help to reveal your emotional state, and help you to deal with it. By examining your intention and attention, you can pinpoint where your mind goes off track. **You can observe where your *attention* is incompatible with your *intention*.** Simply focusing on two simple words like these can enhance cognitive awareness, because they force you to pay attention to incompatible thoughts and emotions.

Intention and attention can also serve the previous exercise. By examining your general intention and you current attention, you may also find it much easier to be able to "frame, name and claim" your current emotional circumstance.

Addressing Past Behaviour

When you look back on particular past events, you can regard them with less attachment. This can also serve the purpose of 'framing.' Using the terms 'intention' and 'attention' while addressing past behaviours can also help frame them.

If you practice these exercises, you will no longer dwell on unwanted food issues or behavioural outcomes; instead, you will focus on what *drives* them. By recalibrating your mindset, you infiltrate and decrease the power any indulgent food issue has over you. You will certainly increase awareness, your capacity for self-restraint, and your response-inhibition. You become more self-aware, as what you focus on expands. I have had clients achieve this without even realizing they were doing it. Yet these were the exact tools they used to eliminate their indulgent food issues.

It's a simple awareness exercise, but it does require diligence and repetition. You cannot just do it once and say "Well, that didn't work." Remember you are trying to deal with *years* of habitual, unconscious reactions. The good news is that since the exercise is so simple, it is also simple to repeat.

Look at past instances where food issues arise. Examine what stimuli—environmental, circumstantial or situational—trigger the unwanted result. Sometimes it is nothing more than a surplus of daily stimuli. Something as simple as this can be enough to create a habitual response to trigger the food issue, so that you may pause the inflow of hyper-stimulation. Noise, crowds and traffic for instance, can all cause stress, and stress-avoidance is often an emotional trigger for eating.

Conversely you may find the opposite to be true. You may be a person who responds well to hyper-stimuli. For you, the old saying "idle minds are the devil's workshop" may be more fitting. For many people, food issues play out as a response to boredom or being alone. Examining past behaviours can help you pinpoint exactly where your triggers have the most power.

Finally, remember that actions result from a sequence of events. The diet and fitness industries want people to think simplistically that:

behaviour —>outcome

But to control and eliminate indulgent food issues requires higher awareness, cognitive awareness.

This is more akin to the equation:

thoughts/feelings —> behaviour/action —>
outcome/experience

Until you develop and exercise some form of higher awareness, your issues will continue. Diet industry gurus want you to believe that "behaviour modification" is the answer. In essence they want you to believe that behaviour determines the mindset, and that if you simply change your behaviour (i.e. follow their diet) then your mind will adapt. But everyone knows what they 'should' eat. So, behaviour modification is only a tiny sliver of the solution. These issues are about *mindset*, and they are *emotional* issues. This is what *drives* the unwanted behaviours.

Chapter 11.
Five Steps to Food Freedom

The Five Steps to Food Freedom are:

1) Structure
2) Regimentation
3) Routine/Rules
4) Choice
5) Freedom

For many people reading this, these steps must be taken in sequence before you can ever rid yourself of unwanted food or eating issues. For others, this sequence will look a lot like the very "diet" sequence that actually caused their issues.

But at some point, self-regulation means taking control of your life *beyond defining it through food and diets.* At some point self-regulation means having an established system in place, where you own your food issue and it no longer owns you.

Committing to a *diet* is an external vehicle of *self-measurement.* Committing to *yourself* is an internal vehicle of *self-expression.* If you do not have the freedom of self-expression, then you may find yourself locked in a diet-prison.

1. Structure

Structure in this case means setting rules. These rules, however, are *not* dominated by diet restrictions. The diet-focus should never be on what foods are not allowed. Instead, focus on food awareness and diet *allowances.*

Over time, structure can help you override impulsivity, but only with the right mindset; **once again the difference is the mental emphasis.** What I mean is a

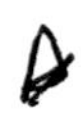

prepared and *planned* response to food cues and environmental stimuli.

The five steps practiced together create a path to self-regulation through self-awareness. This is very different from the usual approach of attaching diet-structure to the mindset of self-denial and self-deprivation.

Having *some form* structure in place for diet, meals and food is backed by ample research in terms of successful outcomes. Regimens that seem totally separate from longterm diet success are actually found to be successful. For instance, research shows that "meal replacement" drinks or powders work, not because of their ingredients or calorie count, **but because they provide structure to meal times and intervals**.

There are tons of data proving that meal regularity is an important element of weight control success. This has as much to do with meal times as well as the actual food on the plate (see Westenhoefer 2004).

2. Regimentation

and

3. Rules

In these cases, but not all, structure and regimentation can seem like just another diet imposed from the outside. Often diet structure can even go as far as dictating what to eat and how much at each particular meal.

How much of this kind of regimentation is necessary will depend on the person and the intensity of the problem. Diet structure and regimentation is only a part of the solution. They are put in place while dealing with other elements of the triangle of awareness.

As food awareness and cognitive awareness build, fewer restrictions are needed, and the rules begin to be followed from the inside out. At first it can be imposed from an external source, like a commitment to a diet, or to a diet coach, until you develop awareness and reach the choice phase. Then, regimentation and rules no longer feel like restriction, but empowered choice. Of course this only happens when previous food issues lose their emotional power and influence over you.

So structure and regimentation are actually a stepping stone along the path to diet freedom.

Usually structure and regimentation surrounding 'a diet' is all about following scripts of denial and deprivation. But rules that are based in a sequence of thought more so than a sequence of behaviour allow you to entertain a different response to the cues that trigger your specific indulgent food issue. In this sense "rules" are not the same as willpower. All willpower does is reinforce the energy of 'attempting resistance' which is emotionally exhausting.

Rules associated with structure and regimentation need to be more cognitively based than behaviourally based. This is what is meant by the term, "mindset determines behaviour."

Think about it—people for whom rules for eating are cognitively based are more positively connected to behavioural choice. This is important. Diet structure, regimentation and rules for these people are not approached from a negative mindset which is focused on externals. That would be the mindset of deprivation and denial. Deprivation and denial only entice emotional provocation which engages the whole futile exercise of willpower. But people who are internally empowered by their diet structure and regimentation are not conflicted. There is no willpower to consider.

4. Choice

Consider someone who becomes a vegetarian for moral, socio-political or environmental reasons. No one imposes this choice. They simply eschew a specific category of food. For these vegetarians, no emotional energy is spent resisting meat, because it is simply not desired.

This is the empowerment of *choice.*

This can work the same way in terms of habit-reversal and letting go of any indulgent food or weight issues. The brain's cognitive power is used to form strong opinions regarding the stimulus. In the vegetarian example, cognition might sound like this: "Factory-farmed animals live a cruel, demeaning existence caused partly by a perversion of government power and capitalist interests, and that wreaks havoc on the environment both locally and abroad. I refuse to take part in that process. I might not be able to stop it, but I can choose not to engage in it."

Nowhere does the above example suggest, "But meat sure would taste good, just this once!"

When I first met my wife she was a meat lover. For a couple of years we frequented a certain chop house because of their meat selection. She would order a filet mignon *and* a pork chop for her 'cheat day.' Years later, researching one of my MP3 nutrition projects. I asked her to read a few of my sources, not thinking much of it at the time. Later that year we went on vacation in Europe. Now, the European outdoor markets are much different urs. Skinned-goats and rabbits hung out in the open.

Knowing what she did about the slaughter process in North America from having read my research materials, as we toured that open market in Croatia, my wife decided then and there to stop eating animal flesh. She became a vegan that day and never looked back. She has not been tempted to eat meat, fish, poultry or dairy since that moment—a moment that transformed her in an instant.

My wife made a *moral* choice, on a higher level of cognitive awareness and association. She didn't do it to lose weight or to look better.

This is known as a **critical perceptual shift.** From that moment, meat had no reward value for her, ever again. Her rules, structure and regimentation about food changed in an instant. But because her change was one of "choice" she felt empowered.

Revisiting Structure

The value of establishing structure, regimentation and rules in order to discard your diet dilemma cannot be underestimated. As a means to freedom from food issues, Robert Jeffrey, PHD, Professor of Epidemiology put it this way:

> *"Giving people specific rules and telling them they are required to follow them as part of their treatment is better than teaching them about the principles of energy balance."*

(By energy balance he means calories, carbs, and fats.)

Jeffrey agrees with me that the pervasiveness of information is practically useless. He also witnesses that, "people tend to abandon structure over time." Therefore structure, regimentation and rules must *lead somewhere*, beyond any type of low-carb, low fat, or macronutrient portioning or restriction.

With this in mind, when it comes to emotional choice and reward value, consider this: when you find yourself before an extravagant buffet, do you home in on all the offerings that *don't* appeal to you? Or, when considering a vacation, do you research all the places where you *don't* want to go?

The goal is to become not just cognitively aware, but more emotionally aware as well. This dual element of self-rebuilding is a process. The goal is to eradicate indulgent food issues by ultimately creating a critical and lasting perceptual shift.

The 5 steps create a process: a process that is non-linear, and allows a person to proceed at his or her own pace and level of awareness.

What is right for you?

Regimentation in the beginning of the process can certainly be helpful, but for others it will exacerbate the problem. This always requires professional assessment in my opinion.

For example, for some people, becoming more diet-regimented only increases the reward value for the problematic foods. The heightened awareness of the specific food craving combined with diet-induced hunger, intensifies desire for the very foods one is trying to avoid. For many people the floodgates open at this point and once they start eating, they're powerless to stop.

In this case, regimentation is the issue. I will discuss this further below.

Establishing an eating routine and sticking to it can be an essential part of regimentation as well. Many people with various food or eating issues witness these issues run amok when they abandon their diet routine.

I have had many clients who write me with similar stories where they are fine on their diets during the week because of structured work hours, and routine, but once they get to the weekends where the routine is disrupted, their eating issues kick in. Sleeping in, running errands and staying up late frequently lead to diet sabotage.

Many people do not realize that "routine" applies not just to a day, but to a whole cycle of days. I usually advise my clients whose problems occur when routines are disrupted, to just stay on their routine. For instance, instead of sleeping in, I advise them to get up at their usual time, and perform their usual routine. If they want to go back to bed after that, they may. However, by then the comfort of their daily routine has been set in motion, instead of thrown off from the beginning.

Little things like this can make all the difference over time. Routine can even be applied to off-schedule meals or eating out. Creating a "date night" and sticking to it can go a long way to keeping people regimented and structured on the other days of the week. For anyone with the indulgent issues we have discussed, structure, regimentation and routine may be the very steps to freedom—even though they seem like backsliding at first.

Diet-structure and routine equals less food chaos in the short- and long-term.

When Should You Count Calories?

I have somewhat vilified the idea of "counting calories" throughout my books and writing. This is because usually it comes from a certain mindset that thinks it can "out-calculate" the human body, or a mindset that is effectively still in a diet prison of some sort. (See my article about whether a calorie is a calorie at: http://scottabelfitness.com/a-calorie-is-a-calorie-um-not/)

There *are* times when it be necessary to at least track calories for a certain period of time.

The reason for this is simple: because many people can no longer accurately feel hunger and satiation.

A restaurant meal may "feel" like 500 calories when in actuality it is well over 1,000. Restaurants are not responsible for your food choices. However, restaurants will definitely take advantage of your conflicting desires.

Case in point: Applebee's is currently advertising a meal menu where each plate is guaranteed to be less than 550 calories. This seems like a great marketing tool. However if you watch the television commercial, you'll see that there's more going on. While the announcer tells you about a menu option where each choice is less than 550 calories, the image is a table with food, wine and beer. Of course these extras are not included in the under 550 calories menu. Most eating establishments know their primary goal is just to get you in the door. From there, your own conception of calorie intake is entirely up to you.

Until a person can reclaim a sense of "justified hunger," counting calories can be a helpful tool. But I want to stress that while for many people counting calories feels like a means of control, for many other people counting calories will feel like an extension of the mindset of diet-prison. **It is always the mindset behind the action that will reveal its usefulness or futility.**

Part of establishing a routine should be a simple rule to never eat outside of meal times. This is a rule everyone should practice. We've already learned that structured meal times were one of the key unconscious weight control mechanisms of our predecessors. *Let's use that.*

This is one simple rule that can help you control weight and lead to better overall health. The beauty and power of this rule is its simplicity. Keep rules and routines simple and intimate, not complex and external. But even though the rules you adapt need to be intimate, keep them non-emotional as well.

As an example, you don't think and worry about a "rule" to brush your teeth or shower on a daily basis. But I am willing to bet that you do in fact brush your teeth or bathe around the same time every day, as part of a routine. And this routine has an unconscious daily ritual and therefore "rule" attached to it. But you don't fret about it. It's not a source of anxiety like the peanut butter jar is for some people.

As a tactic, then, you can set up your own food and diet rules and routines.

Just keep in mind they must be sustainable, and they should be simple. And whenever possible they should avoid conflicts such as pass/fail, good/bad, guilt/reward, and so on.

The "Have To" Mindset

No one likes being told what to do. As an adult, believing you "have to" do anything can produce a sense of justified rebellion.

When clients with eating issues sign up for coaching, part of the package they receive is an instruction manual for eating—not a diet—that comes with an actual sample menu with plenty of options for customization. Many clients perceive this as a 'diet' they are forced follow, so they rebel, usually unconsciously. Often they do not even understand why. They *want* the instruction at the time. They sought it out and paid for it.

Beware: The "have to" mindset will negate every one

of the five steps to Food freedom.

The "have to" mindset disconnects from and rejects the self. A "want to" mindset, if you will, makes cognitive awareness possible, and it embraces and engages the self. This mindset is the foundation for the five steps to food freedom.

The "have to" mindset will often sabotage additional health and fitness strategies as well. When I encounter it as a coach, I know it must be dealt with first and foremost.

One method is to explain and discuss the merits of work ethic and reward. The mindset that leads to rebellion cannot be met with a challenge or more rules. It must be weakened with logic. Any hint of punishment only creates more rebellion, much like a teenager who climbs out his bedroom window when he's been grounded.

I have had many clients come to me after years of working with former trainers who employed punitive methods that only reinforced their "have to" mindsets.

Instead of punishment, understanding and cognitive association can weaken a client's rebelliousness. When a parent raises her teenager to realize that his privileges must be earned; when he learns the value of work firsthand and thereby reaps the results of his labours, he enjoys a new level parental trust and maybe a relaxation of other rules. He also earns the gift of accountability. He now knows that it is he who creates his emotional wealth or poverty—not anyone else enforcing restrictive rules.

It is the attitude of engagement that weakens the defensive mindset of a client who views "diet" as a punishment. They need to be able to connect a *value* to their efforts, and their efforts to a reward. Eventually they will approach their diet structure with an empowered attitude of "want to." This shift takes patience, counselling and experience from a qualified coach.

From Diet Consciousness to Food Awareness

It is first, last and always the mindset *behind* the implementation of the Five Steps that matter most. The goal is to engage individuals so they can connect with themselves and achieve a higher level of cognitive awareness. At some point *behaviour* will change as well.

As I have argued throughout this project, these are awareness issues, not diet-knowledge issues. Part of higher awareness is being cognizant of your own inner strengths. It is about being engaged and connected, not disconnected with self-denial and self-deprivation.

In a recent workshop, I implemented the following checklist, where I used the terms "I-factor" and "Deny-Factor" to illustrate the difference between lower and higher forms of awareness. Lower awareness (mental energy) is likely to be overwhelmed by emotional influences, while higher awareness is less likely to be influenced by emotion.

Use the checklist below to assess your place on the Food Freedom spectrum:

I-Factor:

- Own it
- Forward process
- Do extra work without being asked
- Love the process
- Appreciate where you are and how you got there
- Make the best out of what's given (lemons with lemonade)
- Inspirational
- Gratitude attitude
- Curious and self-investigative
- Caring and devoted
- Zeal for the job at hand
- Awake and engaged
- Do the work for the sake of doing

Deny-Factor:

- Victimized; need validation
- Marching in place
- Do 'what it takes' with no vision
- Need immediate results
- Tolerate requirements
- Endure (lemons are lemons are lemons)

- Seek motivation externally
- Resentful
- Intimidated by change
- Self-absorbed and egocentric
- Wind-up-doll
- Trance-like follower
- Do for the work only for pay off

Where do you see yourself in the checklist? Are you attuned and positive? Are you on track? Is there anything that made you wince with painful recognition? What do you need to address? How can you improve your disposition in order to achieve your goals and ultimate Food Freedom?

Chapter 12.
Behaviour Modification

The behaviour modification (or "B-mod") approach to eradicating or changing unwanted behaviour goes back decades. Its pioneer was B.F. Skinner. (See Skinner, *About Behaviourism*, 1974 for one of the real key works in this field.)

The behavioural method for changing undesired behaviour involves making many small but sustainable adjustments in eating habits, and thinking habits. These changes need to be exercised on a regular basis.

In terms of diet and food this means balanced diets that go easy on fats and sugar. It *doesn't* mean eliminating macronutrients like carbohydrates. That would be severe and drastic, not gradual and balanced.

In terms of behaviour modification external goals like weight loss should be modest and *realistic.* Remember the ultimate goal is cognitive awareness. Essential behaviour modification when it comes to food and eating focuses on sustainable, *permanent* habits, rather than short term strict diet rules.

One of the corollaries of this is that *how* you overcome eating, diet or food issues is less important than *why* you do it. Internal shifts in awareness are more important than any kind of short term behaviour modification, such as 'avoiding carbs.'

But make no mistake: conquering indulgent food issues requires a change in *behaviour.*

A study in the 2005 Journal of the American Medical Association found it was a balanced diet of protein, carbs, and fats that achieved the highest level of diet adherence after one year. Forget about vogue diet trends, pills, potions, cleanses, supplements and complicated mathematical formulas—simple solutions are the most viable, and always have been. This is because they are the easiest to sustain. The problem is that people continue to remain unrealistic about what is possible, and what is sustainable in terms of both eating behaviour and body image.

Mass-marketed programs fail when it comes to offering a full range of behavioural techniques, because eating behaviours are personal and individual. Behaviour modification must be customized; what works for me may not work for you. Yet we see such advice all the time: "Don't eat before bed." "Always eat breakfast." "Never skip a meal," and on and on. These B-mod precepts contain zero regard for context.

We've all heard this one: "Don't eat carbs after 6:00 pm." Well, I have had clients who worked the graveyard shift try not to eat from six o'clock in the evening until six the next morning. Six o'clock PM for someone on the graveyard shift is not six o'clock PM for someone who wakes up at the break of dawn.

However, there is some reasonable generalized advice out there, so let's not throw the baby out with the bathwater. Food writer Michael Pollan, for example, summed up the solution to the modern diet dilemma in seven words: **"Eat food, not a lot, mostly plants."**

It is simple.

It is direct.

And yet is can still be customized and personalized.

It is one of the most effective mantras for behaviour modification to put in someone's mind to begin to alter their cognitive perception. Because it is easy to remember, memorize and repeat, it can have cognitive power as well.

Your own adapted diet rules may indeed follow a general premise but you also need food rules that are personal to you. The rules, like Pollan's instruction above, need to be simple and easy to follow. Part of diet-structure should eventually include variety, but still retain a degree of predictability.

Essential behaviour modification can begin this simple rule: **eat at regular times.**

Here's how it can help you:

1. Eating at regular times eliminates between-meal snacks. As we know, snacking has become the cultural norm, yet for most people it is maladaptive and contributes to weight gain. Meal structure was common practice for generations across cultural divides, and accounted for unconscious, effortless weight control. Inherently, it prevented any kind of consideration of snacking, which meant dealing with and accepting hunger until meal time arrived.

(Please note that snacking on wholesome food still counts as snacking behaviour.)

2. Not snacking leads to another B-mod reminder: **"eat without distraction."** Eating without distraction refers to eating with mindfulness, not counting calories. For example, do not eat while driving, do not eat with the TV on, or while working at the computer. Do not "grab something on the go." Instead, learn to savour.

3. This B-mod is customizable. YOU pick the times that are regular for you and fit into your lifestyle, rather than having to cram yourself into someone else's diet dogma.

Notice also that the rules for consideration of behaviour modification that I condone have less to do with a diet approach and more to do with a food connection. This is important in terms of the mindset awareness which must be positively attached to any changes in behaviour.

One more B-mod approach is: **put your fork down between bites. Chew and swallow your current mouthful before picking up your fork again.** Mindless eating leads to speed eating

These are *simple* behaviour modifications that lead to unconscious weight control and sound eating habits.

Get Some Satisfaction

In terms of actual diet approaches there are some B-mod consideration to make here as well.

Part of any sustainable structured diet solution has to be to **choose foods that satisfy you.** Categorizing foods as permitted or forbidden based on criteria including low carb, low glycemic index, etc., needlessly complicates an initially sound diet structure. Please remember to choose whole foods instead of indulgent junk food.

In terms of sustainable B-mod techniques, the research is clear that eliminating entire food groups from your diet seldom works long-term. Just watch any physique competitor in the post-contest period. Many who eschew all carbs experience the most profound weight gain. Remember the diet-mentality is too often the problem. B-mods lead to long-term success when they reject diet-mentality and emphasize food awareness.

Even healthy foods can be personally enjoyable and

satisfying. Make this a food rule for yourself. From there, **choose foods that you can easily control in terms of portion size and limitation.** If you have any doubt regarding your ability to control a certain food in your diet, then simply eliminate it.

There is an expression in the Tao Te Ching that says, "Frying a fish is spoiled with too much poking." Please don't allow your desire for immediate results thwart the very solutions that with time and space will reveal themselves, and provide results that can last a lifetime. Let your fish fry.

This intelligent attention does not mean focusing on current diet trends that dictate what "should" satisfy you, or foods that are deemed as being "special." Once again these are "externals." They need not mandate your *choices* (remember "choice"? It's step 4 of the Five Steps to Food Freedom.)

If a baked potato satisfies you, but Greek Yogurt does not, then you go with the baked potato. Don't fall for vogue trends that seduce you away from the more satisfying food *for you.* If you like carrots, then eat them. Forget all the nonsense that they're high on the glycemic index. *They're carrots!*

Intelligent B-mod approaches don't follow fads. If your food choice is a wholesome, unprocessed, non-commercially produced food, you're off to great start.

What do YOU crave?

Another way to personalize and individualize your diet plan is to **thoroughly and subjectively examine the types of foods you crave.** This is an internal source cue, instead of an external dictation.

Consider these foods in terms of flavors and textures. Maybe you like crunchy foods, or perhaps you prefer creamy fare. These are texture preferences. In terms of flavors, maybe, like me, you crave sweets—suger. Carbohydrates. Or you could desire the opposite—prime rib or steak or pizza. This denotes a fat preference. If you are diligent with your investigation, you will likely find a common denominator.

Now select whole, unprocessed foods with similar textures, flavors and mouth-feel to those foods you crave. Include these in your diet. Put another way, if you crave chocolate or baked goods, you are not likely to last long on a low carbohydrate diet. Your body communicates with you. Let it guide you. Listen closely.

Get Real & Eat What You Crave

Many women tell me they are 'carb resistant,' even though there is no scientific basis for any such condition. This is an external concept that's been marketed to a specific demographic. These women avoid all carbs, which invariably causes carb cravings, which result in succumbing and finally overeating carbohydrates. Bloating or weight gain results. Is it any wonder they conclude, "I am carbohydrate resistant!" This is a spurious claim, based in circular logic.

It's time to stop pretending that you'll never again eat a particular food, and it's definitely time to stop being ashamed of yourself if you do. Forge a connection between food and *positive* experiences.

Your body is always your keenest source of awareness. One B-mod that may help you step away from diet-consciousness is to **eat what you crave**.

Does that mean if you crave chocolate then chocolate should be included in a behaviour modification approach to alleviating your food issues?

Well, yes and no.

If you examine the components of the chocolate, you will notice a few things, namely a combination of sugar, fat and texture. So someone who craves chocolate would probably benefit from a diet-structure with a specific texture, that is composed of carbohydrates and a little fat. These are the chemical constituents of chocolate. So, that sweet fruit you've been avoiding, or that baked potato you think is forbidden? If you crave chocolate, these foods might just satisfy you. (P.S. White potatoes are wonderful sources of vitamins and minerals and need not be avoided!)

What about the indulgent food itself? Believe it or not, sometimes it is wise to include these foods as part of establishing regular, structured and routine behaviour.

Let's examine the "chocolate lover" above. In fact, let's examine two:

Chocolate lover #1 decides to avoid eating chocolate.

She tries to resist its sweet allure and wills herself to abstain. Eventually, she winds up bingeing on chocolate. (You might be nodding your head in agreement.) The binge leaves her disgusted with herself, which leads her to proclaim, "I'm never eating chocolate again!"

Chocolate lover #2 decides to eat just a little bit of chocolate every day at roughly the same time. She satisfies her craving, knowing she'll have another taste the following day. She gets on with her work, and doesn't think about chocolate for the rest of the day.

Chocolate lover #2 chose an empowered B-mod, which diluted her desire. Usually, people who believe they can't live without the food they crave are mistaken. Confusion is cultivated when we avoid the very foods we adore. Emotional reward value skyrockets. We become obsessed. If we abstain, we're still obsessed, but deprived. If we indulge, we remain obsessed and hate ourselves. So in terms of behaviour modification, tiny daily allowances undermine the value of the emotional reward.

A Note for Food Addicts

Alcohol, street drugs, sleeping pills, anti-depressants, painkillers, nicotine, caffeine, sex, pornography, pain, gambling, social media, television—multitudinal addictions exist and flourish. And additional addictions seem to get discovered and diagnosed every day.

In a world with more leisure time and easy access to almost anything you desire, addiction is predictable and understandable. Those addicted to Facebook have a sort of stimulus addiction. The same can be said of food. We also must remember that food is now produced for a hyper-stimulus effect. Food literally has the power to alter the opioid centres of the brain.

Now, food and eating issues of the modern diet dilemma are one thing. But a food *addiction* or a food *obsession* is another thing altogether. There is a difference between being seduced by a certain food, and being addicted to it.

A food addiction needs to be properly diagnosed and addressed. Because in terms of behaviour modification the cure for a specific food addiction is the same as it is for any other addiction: abstinence from that specific food. Some people may not be sure if they are a food addict or not, or at least addicted to a certain kind of food.

Certain foods exert a magical pull on susceptible individuals. These foods cannot be controlled in terms of portion size or eating behaviour; rather they will be consumed until the sufferer is painfully full and sick.

This is no different than an alcoholic who is unable to stop drinking after one glass. The parallels are well-documented. There is indeed such a thing as a food addiction. If someone has a legitimate chocolate addiction, for example, then the above scenario regarding the chocolate lover who indulges just a little bit every day would not be recommended, nor would it work.

Addiction is a physiological disease, far more serious (and deadly in some cases) than modern indulgent food issues. Moreover, the troublesome thing about genuine food addiction is that it is so hard to pinpoint and it causes less obvious physical damage.

An Extreme Experiment

Let me first explain how and why I began conducting this experiment. Additionally I must note that I *only* advise this on *very rare* occasions.

I once had a client who believed she couldn't live without chocolate. No matter what I said, she asserted that her weakness for chocolate was not like anyone else's. She was convinced it was some sort of metabolic glitch or food addiction.

I disagreed.

The more I tried to explain otherwise, the deeper her conviction grew. But this client also knew that her so-called addiction was undermining physique goals. So I employed a little reverse psychology. I instructed to *live on nothing but chocolate for five days.* All she was permitted to eat was her favourite type of chocolate, and water. I gave her no additional rules regarding calories control or portion control. Before she even started she worried about how much weight she would gain, because she was sure she would binge the whole week.

By late afternoon on day two, she was already growing weary of chocolate. By the third and fourth days she was begging me to let her go back to her diet. For weeks after the experiment, she couldn't look at or think about chocolate.

So much for the idea that she physically "needed" it. This proved to her that her convictions regarding chocolate were pure, misguided fantasy. And yet for years she had endured a self-fulfilling prophecy because she believed she "needed" chocolate every day.

A male client who was convinced he "needed" pasta experienced the same result. .

After this experiment neither client ever suffered issues with either food ever again.

You can implement this experiment for yourself to find out if you have a food addiction. You must commit to eating nothing but the suspected food for three to five days, and no fluids except for water. If your addiction is specifically to *butter pecan* ice-cream you must eat that flavour for the duration. If your presumed addiction is chocolate then choose the most mouth-watering variety.

If after a few days the thought of eating more of your assigned food makes you queasy or upset, then you can discontinue the experiment. You are not "addicted," but merely seduced by it (or at least you used to be). It is a trigger food for maladaptive behaviour and nothing more. The allure you experienced was not physical, but entirely in your mind.

However, if you find that by the end of the experiment this food *still* appeals to you, you more than likely do have a food addiction. If this is the case, then abstinence will be the healthiest choice, along with an evaluation from a qualified addiction specialist.

Behavioural modification techniques are educational tools meant to be used and applied to enhance awareness. Remember that behaviours are skills, and they can be learned with regular practice. Also know that these are meant to be subjective, positive experiences.

Any techniques used should eventually combine mental and emotional awareness as well. Behaviour modification can be assigned as both a means and eventually an ends to eradicating unwanted eating issues.

Chapter 13. Freedom

The modern diet dilemma will not be solved with a bigger microscope, but rather a bigger macroscope.

We are the same species we were in the 1970s. But the 1970s saw the business of eating change radically when for the first time, farming became profit-driven, commodity crops exploded with surplus and mammoth corporate farms unfurled across the American landscape. The market usurped subsistence as well as sustenance. The result shows on our bodies as so many of us grow ever more malnourished, hungry and overweight.

We are fed what marketers want us to believe. Our current environment is one in which sophisticated, suppressive and omnipresent marketing efforts prey on every one of our food and diet choices. Marketing preys on our desires for sensory gratification; on the ease with which we accept misinformation. Then corporate interests deliver the goods—products to help us feel better, look better, and "be" better.

The truth is almost everybody who tries to "diet" to lose weight will fail in the long run. In 2007, *The American Psychological Association* reviewed 31 different diet studies. What they found shouldn't surprise us: after two years, over two-thirds of dieters ended up weighing MORE than they did before they started their diets. In fact, the more frequently someone "diets," the more difficult it becomes to lose weight—and the easier it becomes to gain weight—over time. This hardly sounds like a winning formula or a solution. It is clear that dieting is part of the problem. Yet the myth continues.

Yet, in our current culture of abundance and entitlement, we love to believe in neat fixes. The "unbiased" media accommodate us by playing up "new research findings" in one headline after another, as if they're viable solutions or absolutes. And the studies most likely to grab media attention are the ones that offer up scientific-sounding solutions and cater to our emotions. But if you look closely, you'll find that these findings conflict with one another, or are merely suggestive of an idea. Hasn't this been the modus operandi for decades now? So why are we still struggling?

A study in last September's *American Journal of Clinical Nutrition*, for example, found a link between increased dairy intake and weight loss. However, a meta-analysis in the May 2008 *Nutrition Review* yielded no link. A paper in the *Journal of Occupational and Environmental Medicine* from January 2010 proposed a connection between job stress and obesity. However, in October of 2010, a report in the journal *Obesity* concluded there was no such correlation.

On the micro scale, your habits are shaped by the eating and thinking habits of your friends and acquaintances. We actually model what we see most often, not what we are told, or what we "know." On the macro scale, the food industry wields a strong influence through its marketing, and in the production of hyper-palatable food products. In terms of changing our environment, we must focus whenever possible on micro and macro influences that impact us in positive, productive ways, because the effect of such cunning mass marketing along with interpersonal social cues, is that eating habits become modelled, contagious behaviours—the common cold of eating issues.

There *are* solutions.

YOU, the dieter, and not the diet—are now the focus of your personal diet dilemma. Beyond being personal, practical and empowering, your diet strategy needs to be realistic, reasonable and sustainable.

Cognitive Restructuring

Your ultimate goal is empowerment. This is *not* the same as positive thinking. This kind of awareness means assuming control of your thoughts and your reaction to your thoughts.

You develop higher awareness by paying attention to your thought patterns, the situation that preceded them and the conditions surrounding them. Pay *less* attention to the behavioural results. Your behaviour does not define you, even if you believe it has for a long time. Once you accomplish this level of awareness, you define your own behaviour, without the conflict or energy of 'willpower.'

This is the cognitive shift required; nothing more and nothing less will eradicate whatever issues you suffer from. With practice, you arrive at a point where your issues hold no power. The anxiety-provoking thoughts may arise momentarily, but soon dissolve into the ether like smoke.

This is a journey, not a destination. You realize as you travel that your food and eating issues are not a battle you fight, but confusion you meet with understanding. That's when they let you go.

Make no mistake, habit-reversal takes time. The process is never linear. You cannot "force" awareness. You can only develop it, like you would a muscle or a reading skill. You can never accomplish this by ignoring the issues, or resisting them. Awareness is something you must invite into your consciousness. Looking at it in this way, your residual struggles become opportunities for growth rather than terrible burdens to be endured.

The physical, mental and emotional realms of experience are connected, even if you don't realize it. This means you can never just "think" your way to awareness. Dare to feel and address your emotior and discomfort are requisite but temporary. The only way you can ever be 'ready' for that challenge is to just immerse yourself in it.

Emotionally and mentally you are only successful when your dilemma becomes a non-issue. This means that food no longer holds emotional power, and doesn't take up any mental space during your day.

This is what true freedom from food and diet issues actually is. Headlong through the storm is the only way out. This freedom is, in essence, the ability to eat normally with no preoccupation with food one way or another.

The successful mindset is one of self-mastery; the behavioural emphasis is secondary.

This is what most people seem to miss. At all my workshops I give at least one lecture on self-mastery. Some attendees are unable to relate: "Self-mastery? What does that have to do with getting ready for a bodybuilding competition?"

Yet self-mastery is connected to each and every endeavour in life. It's about understanding that it's not the recipe, but the mastery of the chef that ensures a distinctive dish. Everyone wants recipes to follow. Few want to put in the required efforts to becoming the chef.

I tell attendees every year that Fortune 500 companies pay millions of dollars for guest speakers and company retreats, all for the purpose of nurturing higher awareness and self-mastery. In terms of food issues, self-mastery means knowing and embracing the concept of choice. Once emotion is removed from the equation there is no longer an issue. The revelation is that there never really was an issue. You realize that your issue was never about food at all, but your attitude toward it.

You need to embrace your own empowerment, not your perceived entitlement, and certainly not your perceived victimhood. You do not have a "food" or "diet" or "weight" issue. Those issues are external to you, and because they are external to you, you exercise no power over them. Perceiving your own emotional reception as a dial you turn like the volume on your car stereo means you control the settings.

In terms of the macroscopic environment, you can control that as well. Utilize your exposure to food, fitness and supplement marketing. Question it. Analyze it. Research it. Debate it. This will weaken its emotional appeal. It will also weaken your tendency to react first and think later. Your practiced awareness will come to encompass the flaccid reality behind industry hype. They want your money—not your wellness. Why? Because true wellness is your responsibility. No one has the power to market something you already own.

Do not discount the power of marketing. It's expertly designed to appeal to any emotional need you have. Taste, convenience, health, personality, popularity, lifestyle and all things in between—it's all fair play. Diligently disarm the marketing power by suspending your disbelief. Pay attention, son.

Instead of allowing marketing to appeal to your

emotional reaction centers, use your own mental of the marketing aimed at you to *respond.* This creates cognitive disruption and reduces the potential power of the marketing message. Understand straight away that none of these industries ever presents you with "neutral" information. And dial down your emotional response.

As you begin to solve your own issues you will more than likely experience a **"critical perceptual shift"** (as with the vegetarian who never craves meat again). This means you come to see yourself and the world around you in an entirely different and new light. (The term was originally employed by doctors Ludwig and Litman, who treat alcoholism. See References.) For people with indulgent food or eating issues, a permanently changed perception regarding food is the final element of permanent freedom.

The final solution to your own personal modern diet dilemma is one of cognitive restructuring and self-mastery. Notice that the terms used here have nothing to do with carbohydrates, fats, proteins or nutrient timing.

To rid yourself of any and all food and eating issues, make the following acknowledgements:

- You do not commit to a diet. You commit to *yourself.*

- Commitment to a diet is a commitment to an alienating and disempowering external force—one that cultivates internal conflict.

- Committing to yourself develops your awareness

capacity.

- Only once you commit to *yourself* can you commit to a *diet*, which then becomes a process, not a goal.

You do not have a food or eating issue; you have an awareness issue.

Review your answers to the questionnaire. What challenges can you now face head on, right now, after reading this book? Think it over carefully. You can start right now, if you haven't already. Addressing the questions one by one enhances self-awareness. As you progress, additional undesirable elements of your own personal dilemma will tend to fall like dominos.

So: how do you eliminate whatever personal food or diet issue you have? You go back to the beginning!

Key Phrases & Summary Points:

- The modern diet dilemma requires a shift from diet-consciousness to food awareness.
- We have evolved to easily gain and resist losing weight.
- Over 75% of physique competitors, after a two-year period, will weigh more and look "heavier" than they did before they began training for competition.
- Behavioural fixes like "diets" work against our

bodies' natural design, and as such are incomplete.

- Research shows that chronic overeating and its effects create a neural feedback loop with the same biochemical markers of drug addiction.
- Modern diet issues are solved by awareness, not further dieting.
- The focus of your solution must be YOU (the dieter), not the diet.
- Your behaviour does not define you.
- Pain may be necessary in order to end suffering.
- You cannot diet your way to awareness.
- You cannot diet your way out of mental, emotional or biological constraints.
- The real solution to your personal diet dilemma is cognitive restructuring and self-mastery.

References

Barrett, Deidre *Waistland: The (R)evolutionary Science Behind Our Weight and Fitness Crisis* (2007)

Bevins, Rick A., and Michael Bardo, *Motivational Factors in the Etiology of Drug Abuse,* (2004)

Bobroff, E.M., and H.R. Kissileff, "Effects of Changes in Palatability on Food Intake and the Cumulative Food Intake Curve in Man," *Appetite*, 7, #1, (1986)

Brandsma, L.L., "Physician and Patient Attitudes Toward Obesity," *Eating Disorders*, 13, #2, (2005)

Baumeister, R.F., ed. *Handbook of Self-Regulation: Research, Theory and Application* (2004)

Datamonitor, "Soaring Stress Levels Drive British Consumers to Splash Out on Premium Treats" *Datamonitor*, Oct., (2004)

Drewnowski, A., "Energy Intake and Sensory Properties of Food," *American Journal of Clinical Nutrition*, 62, #5, (1995)

Drewnowski, A., and M.R. Greenwood, "Cream and Sugar: Human Preferences for High-Fat Foods," *Physiology and Behavior*, 30, #4 (1983)

Emmett, P.M., and K.W. Heaton, "Is Extrinsic Sugar a Vehicle for Dietary Fat?" *Lancet*, 345, #8964

Ferriday, D. and J.M. Brunston, "How does Food-Cue Exposure Lead to Larger Meal Sizes?" *British Journal of Nutrition* (2008)

Fischer, S., et al, "Coping with Distress by Eating or Drinking: Role of Trait Urgency and Expectancies," *Psychology of Addictive Behavior,* 18, #3, (2004)

Flegal, K.M., and R.P. Troiano, "Changes in the Distribution of Body Mass Index of Adults and Children in the US population," *International Journal of Obesity and Related Metabolic Disorders,* 24, #7 (2000)

Franken, I.H., "The Role of Dopamine in Human Addiction: From Reward to Motivated Attention," *European Journal of Pharmacology*, 526, #'s 1-3, (2005)

Freedman, David H. "How to Fix the Obesity Crisis," in *Scientific American* Volume 304, #2, (2011)

Grigson, P.S., "Like Drugs for Chocolate: Separate Rewards Modulated by Common Mechanisms?" *Physiology and Behavior*, 76, #3, (2002)

Gross, J. ed. *Handbook of Emotion Regulation,* (2007)

Harvey, E.L., and A.J. Hill, "Health Professionals Views of Overweight People and Smokers," *International Journal of Obesity and Related Metabolic Disorders*, 25, #8, (2001)

Heatherton, T.F. and R.F. Baumeister, "Binge Eating as Escape from Self-Awareness," *Psychological Bulletin*, 110, #1, (1991)

James, W.P. "Energy and Macronutrient Needs in Relation to Substrate Handling in Obesity," in *Clinical Obesity in Adults and Children*, 2nd ed. (2005)

Kaplan, L.M., "Body Weight Regulation and Obesity," *Journal of Gastrointestinal Surgery*, 7, #4 (2003)

Keesey, R.E. and M.D. Hirvonen, "Body Weight Set Points: Determination and Adjustment," *Journal of Nutrition*, 127, #9, (1997)

Kessler, David A. *The End of Overeating* (2009)

Kolata, Gina *Rethinking Thin* (2007)

Larson, D.E., et al, "Spontaneous Overfeeding with a Cafeteria Diet in Men: Effects on 24 Hour Energy Expenditure and Substrate Oxidation," *International Journal of Obesity and Related Metabolic Disorders*, 19, #5, (1995)

Macias, A.E., "Experimental Demonstration of Human Weight Homeostasis: Implications for Understanding Obesity," *British Journal of Nutrition*, 91, #3 (2004)

McGuire, M.T., et al, "What Predicts Weight Regain in a Group of Successful Weight Losers?" *Journal of Consulting and Clinical Psychology*, 67, #2, (1999)

Mela, David J., and Peter J. Rogers. *Food, Eating, and Obesity: The Psychobiological Basis of Appetite and Weight Control*, (1998)

Mercer, J.G., and J.R. Speakman, "Hypothalmic Neuropeptide

Mechanisms for Regulating Energy Balance: From Rodents to Human Obesity," *Neuroscience and Biobehavioral Reviews*, 25, #2, (2001)

Mela, D.J., "Eating for Pleasure or Just Wanting to Eat? Reconsidering Sensory Hedonic Responses as a Driver of Obesity," *Appetite*, 47, #1, (2006)

Mitchell, James E., *Binge-Eating Disorder: Clinical Foundations and Treatment*, (2008)

Moore, Judith *Fat Girl* (2005)

Mrdjenovic, G. and D.A. Levitsky, "Children Eat What They are Served: The Imprecise Regulation of Energy Intake," *Appetite*, 44, #3, (2005)

Naleid, A.M., et al, "Deconstructing the Vanilla Milkshake: The Dominant Effect of Sucrose on Self-Administration of Nutrient Flavor Mixtures," *Appetite*, 50, #1, (2008)

Ogden, C.L., et al, "Mean Body Weight, Height, and Body Mass Index, United States, 1960- 2002" *Advanced Data from Vital Health Statistics*, 347 (2004)

Ogden, C.L., et al, "Prevalence and Trends in Overweight among US Children and Adolescents, 1999- 2009" *JAMA*, 14 (2002)

Ogden, C.L., et al, "Prevalence of Overweight and Obesity in the United States, 1999-2004," *JAMA*, 13 (2006)

Pearcey, S.M. and J. M. de Castro, "Food Intake and Meal Patterns of Weight-Stable and Weight-Gaining Persons," *American Journal of Clinical Nutrition,* 76, #1, (2002)

Pinel, John *Biopsychology*, 6th edition, (2007)

Proulx, K. "Experiences of Women with Bulimia Nervosa in a Mindfulness-Based Eating Disorder Treatment Group," *Eating Disorders*, 16, #1, (2008)

Roberts, Paul *The End of Food*, (2008)

Rolls, Edmund T, *The Brain and Emotion*, (1999)

Rolls, Edmund T, "Taste, Olfactory, and Food Texture Processing in the Brain, and the Control of Food Intake," *Physiology and Behavior* 85, #1, (2005)

Schwartz, M.W. and K.D. Niswender, "Adiposity Signaling and Biological Defense Against Weight Gain: Absence of Protection or Central Hormone Resistance?" *Journal of Endocrinology and Metabolism*, 89, #12 (2004)

Shils, Maurice E., et al, eds. *Modern Nutrition in Health and Disease*, 11th edition, (2010)

Siddartha, William, *On Desire: Why We Want What We Want* (2006)

Skinner, B.F. About Behaviorism (1974)

Stunkard, A.J. and S. Messick, "The Three-Factor Eating Questionnaire to Measure Dietary Restraint, Disinhibition, and Hunger," *Journal of Psychosomatic Research*, 29, #1, (1985)

Stunkard, A.J., et al, "Predictors of Body Size in the First 2 Years of Life: A High Risk Study of Human Obesity," *International Journal of Obesity and Related Metabolic Disorders*, 28, #4 (2004)

Wansink, B., et al, "Environmental Factors That Increase the Food Intake and Consumption Volume of Unknowing Consumers," *Annual Review of Nutrition,* 24, (2004)

Wells, Adrian and Gerald Matthews, *Attention and Emotion: A Clinical Perspective,* (1994)

Westenhoefer, J., et al, "Behavioral and Correlates of Successful Weight Reduction over 3 years: Results from Lean Habits Study," *International Journal of Obesity and Related Metabolic Disorders*, 28, #2, (2004)

Wirtshafter, D. and J.D. Davis, "Set Points, Settling Points, and the Control of Body Weight," *Physiology and Behaviour,* 19, #1, (1977)

Wise, R. A. "Brain Reward Circuitry: Insights from Unsensed Incentives," *Neuron*, 36, #2, (2002)

Wise, R. A. "Dopamine and Food Reward: Back to the Elements," *American Journal of Physiology: Regulatory, Integrative and Comparative Physiology,* 286, #1, (2004)

Wise, R.A. "Role of Brain Dopamine in Food Reward and Reinforcement," *Philosophical Transactions of the Royal Society of London: Series B: Biological Sciences*, 361, #1471 (2006)

Yeomans, M.R., "Taste, Palatability and the Control of Appetite," *Proceedings of the Nutrition Society*, 57, #4, (1998)

Yeomans, M.R., et al, "Palatability: Response to Nutritional Need or Need-Free Stimulation of Appetite?" *British Journal of Nutrition,* 92, Supplement 1, (2004)

Learn More

To learn more about diet, mindset, training, and physique transformation, or to get announcements about future books, please visit my website and subscribe to my email list: **scottabelfitness.com**.

I send out free articles on nutrition and working out, as well as case studies, client updates, and more.

If you liked this book, and want to see more, please take a moment to **write a review on Amazon** and let me know!

DISCLAIMER AND/OR LEGAL NOTICES: Every effort has been made to accurately represent this book and it's potential. Results vary with every individual, and your results may or may not be different from those depicted. No promises, guarantees or warranties, whether stated or implied, have been made that you will produce any specific result from this book. Your efforts are individual and unique, and may vary from those shown. Your success depends on your efforts, background and motivation.

The material in this publication is provided for educational and informational purposes only and is not intended as medical advice. The information contained in this book should not be used to diagnose or treat any illness, metabolic disorder, disease or health problem. Always consult your physician or health care provider before beginning any nutrition or exercise program. Use of the programs, advice, and information contained in this book is at the sole choice and risk of the reader

Made in the USA
Monee, IL
04 April 2023

31346159R00108